Yoga and Eating Disorders

Yoga and Eating Disorders bridges the knowledge and practice gaps between mental health providers and yoga practitioners who work with clients suffering from disordered eating. Combining the wisdom of 20 experts in eating disorders treatment and yoga practice, editors Carolyn Costin and Joe Kelly show how and why yoga's mind–body connection facilitates treatment and recovery. This invaluable resource for mental health and yoga professionals, as well as individuals and family members struggling with eating disorders, explores the use of yoga in therapy, ways yoga teachers can recognize and respond to disordered eating, recovery stories, research into yoga's impact on symptoms, and much more.

Carolyn Costin recovered from anorexia in her twenties, became a therapist, and saw her first eating disorder client in 1979. She then developed and directed several inpatient eating disorder facilities. In 1996, Carolyn opened Monte Nido, the first state of the art residential treatment program to bring together Eastern and Western healing modalities, including yoga and meditation. Carolyn left Monte Nido & Affiliates in early 2016 to pursue other passions, while continuing to provide her renowned clinical insight, wisdom and professional training worldwide. Carolyn's books include *The Eating Disorder Source Book, 100 Questions and Answers About Eating Disorders, 8 Keys to Recovery from an Eating Disorder* (companion workbook in press), and *Your Dieting Daughter.* To learn more, visit www.carolyncostin.com and www.yogaandeatingdisorders.com, or email carolyn@carolyncostin.com.

Joe Kelly has been a journalist since 1985, was an award-winning reporter for Minnesota Public Radio, and co-founded *New Moon Girls* magazine and the nonprofit Dads & Daughters. He served on the Eating Disorders Coalition board, and was Fathering Educator at The Emily Program. His 13 books include *Dads & Daughters, The Complete Idiot's Guide to Being a New Dad* and (with Margo Maine, PhD) *The Pressure to Be Perfect: Eating Disorders, Body Myths and Women at Midlife and Beyond.* Joe has contributed chapters to *Prevention of Eating- and Weight-Related Disorders* and *Encyclopedia of Diversity in Education.* Joe trains eating disorder and addiction professionals how to engage clients' male loved ones as treatment and recovery allies. To learn more, visit www.joekelly.org or email joe@joekelly.org.

Yoga and Eating Disorders
Ancient Healing for Modern Illness

Edited by
Carolyn Costin and Joe Kelly

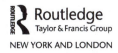

NEW YORK AND LONDON

First published 2016
by Routledge
711 Third Avenue, New York, NY 10017

and by Routledge
2 Park Square, Milton Park, Abingdon, Oxon OX14 4RN

Routledge is an imprint of the Taylor & Francis Group, an informa business

© 2016 Taylor & Francis

Library of Congress Cataloging in Publication Data
Names: Costin, Carolyn, editor. | Kelly, Joe, 1954- editor.
Title: Yoga and eating disorders? : ancient healing for modern illness / edited by Carolyn Costin and Joe Kelly.
Description: New York, NY : Routledge, 2016. |
Includes bibliographical references and index.
Identifiers: LCCN 2015039166 | ISBN 9781138908451 (hbk : alk. paper) | ISBN 9781138908468 (pbk : alk. paper) | ISBN 9781315694405 (ebk)
Subjects: LCSH: Eating disorders--Treatment--Popular works. | Hatha yoga--Popular works.
Classification: LCC RC552.E18 Y64 2016 | DDC 613.7/046--dc23
LC record available at http://lccn.loc.gov/2015039166

ISBN: 978-1-138-90845-1 (hbk)
ISBN: 978-1-138-90846-8 (pbk)
ISBN: 978-1-315-69440-5 (ebk)

Typeset in Sabon
by Taylor & Francis Books

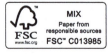

MIX
Paper from
responsible sources
FSC™ C013985

Printed in the United Kingdom
by Henry Ling Limited

Contents

Contributors

Lori Allen, PhD, RYT 200, is a licensed psychologist and certified yoga instructor in Eugene, Oregon. She runs Yoga Mind Psychotherapy, using the art of yoga and science of psychotherapy to treat eating disorders, women's issues, anxiety, depression and trauma. Lori has been a therapist at the University of Oregon Counseling Center and her yoga practice focuses on taking time each day to center, prioritizing what's important and becoming fully ourselves.

Tosca Braun, MA, is a 200-hour Kripalu Yoga instructor and 500-hour Integrative Yoga Therapist. She is also a doctoral student in Clinical Health Psychology at the University of Connecticut, where she conducts research on yoga, mindfulness and health. Tosca spent five years as a research intern and project manager with Kripalu's Institute for Extraordinary Living in Massachusetts, an organization devoted to the scientific study of yoga-based curricula. She holds bachelor's degrees from Reed College and SUNY Empire State College in history and health psychology, respectively, and has more than 2,000 hours of training in yoga, Ayurveda and the mind-body connection.

Julie Carmen, MA, LMFT, ERYT-500, is a Licensed Marriage and Family Therapist and Associate Director of Mental Health at Loyola Marymount University Yoga Therapy Rx. She worked as a yoga therapist at Passages and Monte Nido Eating Disorder Centers and for 12 years taught weekly community classes at the Exhale studio in Venice, California. Julie designed and implemented a yoga therapy program at Los Angeles Unified School District's Pregnant Teens program and worked as a drama therapist at Cell Block Theater in Manhattan. She has small private psychotherapy and yoga therapy practices, is a professional film and stage actor and owns the indie yoga media production company yogatalks.com.

Lisa Diers, RD, LD, E-RYT, is Director of Nutrition Services and Yoga Manager for The Emily Program, which treats eating disorders in Minnesota, Ohio, Pennsylvania and Washington State. She graduated from the University of Minnesota Medical Center/Fairview Hospital/University of

Minnesota Children's Hospital dietetic internship program, and has been a dietitian since 2000. Lisa is passionate about the healing power that both nutrition and yoga provide to those struggling with disordered eating and negative body image.

Nicole Dunas, MFA, is Counseling Intern Practitioner at Noeticus Counseling Center in Denver and pursuing her MA in transpersonal counseling psychology at Naropa University in Boulder, Colorado. She completed a 200-hour yoga instructor training certification and has undergone training in Restorative Justice and safeTALK Suicide Awareness. Nikki is also an enthusiastic writing tutor and passionate writer with an MFA in creative writing from Bennington (VT) College.

Laura Dunn studies Indian religions, yoga traditions, Sanskrit and Hindi at the University of Hawaii, where she is also a graduate teaching assistant completing her Master's in religious studies. She teaches and practices yoga avidly while maintaining her interests in Buddhist philosophy and meditation. Laura enjoys watching the ways in which these practices intersect and unfold in modern everyday life. She is primarily interested in the relevance and meaning of traditional yoga in modernity, and how ascetic practices such as yoga are a gateway to deeper inner and outer knowledge.

David Emerson, E-RYT is Founder and Director of Yoga Services for the Trauma Center at the Justice Resource Institute in Brookline Massachusetts, where he coined the term "trauma-sensitive yoga." He has extensive experience in the instruction of yoga with PTSD in various populations; developing, conducting and supervising yoga groups for rape crisis centers, domestic violence programs, residential programs for youth, military bases, survivors of terrorism and Veterans Administration centers and clinics. David is co-author of *Overcoming Trauma through Yoga* (Berkeley, CA: North Atlantic Books, 2011) and author of *Trauma Sensitive Yoga* (New York: Norton, 2015).

Lori Haas, MSW, LCSW, CEDS, is a holistic oriented psychotherapist in Tempe, Arizona specializing in eating disorders, trauma and anxiety for girls and women. She is also trained in Eye Movement Desensitization and Reprocessing (EMDR) therapy. Lori is a master level (500 Hour) Certified Yoga Teacher and Yoga Therapist specializing in Healing Emphasis Yoga. Her Yoga Healing Groups and workshops focus on opening the heart and being more connected emotionally, physically and spiritually on and off the yoga mat.

Robyn Hussa Farrell, MFA, E-RYT is Founder and CEO of mentalfitness, inc. and an award-winning producer, performer, educator and author. She created eating disorder recovery yoga programs for inpatient and outpatient treatment programs and has offered free recovery yoga to patients in recovery (and their families) for over a decade in Wisconsin,

New York City and Spartanburg, South Carolina. With her husband Tim Farrell, Robyn has co-directed documentary films including *Speaking Out About Ed* and *ED 101*.

Caroline Keating received her yoga training from the Krishnamacharya Yoga Mandiram in Chennai, India and has worked on in-patient treatment teams since 2004. She directed yoga programs for eating disorder and chemical dependency recovery. Caroline's practice is deeply steeped in a personal understanding that the only way out of the labyrinth of mental and health issues is through it. Her life work is to share the healing tools of yoga as well as cultivate a culture of wellness and prevention for future generations. Caroline and her family live on Orcas Island, Washington.

Sarah Lazar, PhD, is director of the meditation research laboratory at Massachusetts General Hospital in Boston and Assistant Professor of Psychology at Harvard University, where she earned her PhD in microbiology. Sara and her team use neuroimaging techniques to study neurological, cognitive, emotional and brain structure changes associated with meditation and yoga practice. She has contributed research articles to numerous scientific journals and her research has been covered by news organizations including *The New York Times, USA Today*, CNN, National Public Radio, WebMD and the Huffington Post.

Melody Moore, PhD, RYT is a Clinical Psychologist, yoga instructor, author, activist and Founder of Embody Love Yoga. She completed a post-doctoral internship at Children's Medical Center of Dallas' Eating Disorder program and her yoga teacher training at the Dallas Yoga Center. After seven years in private practice specializing in eating disorder recovery, Melody chose to combine the healing tools of yoga, embodied experience and psychodynamic therapy to create Embody Love Movement, a program that allows people to know that they are valuable and worthy.

Maria Sorbara Mora, MS, RD, PRYT, RYT is a clinical nutritionist, exercise physiologist, yoga teacher and yoga therapist in New York City. She has a Masters of Science in Nutrition and Applied Physiology from Columbia University and is a Certified Phoenix Rising Yoga Therapy Group Facilitator. Maria has presented on interdisciplinary approaches to eating disorders treatment at professional conferences in the US and Europe, and written for the International Journal of Eating Disorders. She believes that to recover from eating disorders and body issues, one needs to learn to connect to their body as a pathway to healing.

Elisa Mott EdS, NCC, RYT has led therapeutic yoga groups for adults and adolescents at Kaiser Permanente's eating disorder intensive outpatient unit in Walnut Creek, California. She has Masters of Education and Education Specialist degrees in Mental Health Counseling from the

University of Florida, along with a certificate in Spirituality and Health and Arts in Medicine. Elisa writes and presents nationally on the use of yoga in the treatment of eating disorders and body image issues. She teaches yoga in Pleasanton, California.

Joanna O'Neal, E-RYT teaches kids, teens, family and community yoga classes as well as chair yoga classes for seniors in San Diego County, California. She believes that everyone can benefit physically and mentally from yoga, regardless of age, sex, religion, or physical ability. She specializes in Purna Yoga, which focuses on the heart as the center of the self, allowing the practitioner to distinguish between the self of the mind, the true self and deeper wisdom of the heart.

Elyse Parcher, MS, 500-RYT is a therapist for Dine Monte Nido in Ardmore, Pennsylvania. She often integrates yoga into the therapeutic process. Elyse uses deep breathing, meditation, gentle movement, body awareness, mindfulness and yoga philosophy to illuminate the ways in which yoga helped facilitate her own recovery from an eating disorder. She earned her Master's in Counseling and Clinical Health Psychology from the Philadelphia College of Osteopathic Medicine.

Lauren Peterson, E-RYT-500, is a student of Iyengar yoga, and an advanced (fourth series) ashtanga yoga practitioner. Lauren has been featured in the television series Healing Quest and *Yoga Journal* magazine for the yoga program she started for women at the Monte Nido Eating Disorders Center. She created a yoga practice CD "The Yogi's Companion," picked as a *Yoga Journal* "editor's choice." Lauren teaches private and group classes in Malibu, CA; she also teaches ashtanga and vinyasa workshops nationwide.

Tamar Siegel, MA is studying at the Interdisciplinary Center in Herzliya, Israel and plans to complete her PhD in Counseling Psychology at the University of Tel Aviv. Previously, she worked in Dr. Catherine Cook-Cottone's University of Buffalo laboratory researching yoga, mindfulness and eating disorders. Tamar earned an MA in clinical psychology at Columbia University and, to gain a deeper understanding of the healing aspects of yoga, she completed her 200-hour Kripalu yoga teacher training. Combining her personal experience with academic research, Tamar hopes to develop evidence-based treatments for female adolescents that incorporate yoga and mindfulness practices.

Jamie Silverstein, E-RYT 500, CHC, is a registered yoga teacher, certified health counselor and former Olympic athlete. She owns The Grinning Yogi studio in Seattle and facilitates yoga and the body groups at The Eating Disorders Recovery Center of Washington. Jamie's work has been published on the *Yoga Journal*, MindBodyGreen, YogaDork and DoYouYoga websites. She believes that, to quote the Sufi poet Hafiz, the "wounds of love" from an eating disorder can heal and become seeds of strength.

Foreword

Linda Sparrowe

Anyone who walks into a typical yoga class and sees a room full of flexible, lithe bodies moving through multiple sun salutations, kicking up into handstand and then effortlessly landing in a perfect yoga push-up—all the while barely breaking a sweat—can be forgiven for wondering how a practice so obsessed with physical perfection could help her heal a disordered body image. Even if she doesn't stay and endure 90 minutes of comparison shopping (*I want thighs like those! How much yoga do I have to do to look like that? My belly will never be that flat*), she may easily leave feeling worse about herself than when she came in.

How did this ancient spiritual practice morph into a thinly disguised exercise in self-absorption? What happened to its inherent promise of self-reflection and transformation? Alas, as physicality trumped spirituality in the West, yoga became separated from its essential teachings and things began to unravel a bit. We heard yoga's invitation to reflect, but somehow missed the "without judgment" part. We reflect alright, but with unrelenting self-criticism. We loved the transformation part, but only as a way of changing the size and shape of our thighs, necks and bellies. We failed to read the fine print: yoga is not interested in transforming our body; it's interested in transforming our *relationship* to the body we already have, helping us celebrate its usefulness and its beauty.

Yoga's mission is to wake us up to our true selves, to the beauty already within, to move us from separation to connection, from contraction to spaciousness, and from fear to acceptance. How it does that, of course, depends on the needs of the person it serves. Sometimes a strong physical practice is what's called for. Other times, doing a simple pranayama technique will show how regulating the breath can soften intense emotions. Still other times, just sitting and noticing a reluctance to sit and notice—that's yoga, too. For women with eating disorders, the rift between the mind and body has deepened over the years, and the chasm may be too wide to mend easily.

Luckily there are people in the world, like Carolyn Costin, who believe in yoga's ability to restore that fractured relationship—and who have the skills, wisdom and compassion needed to put that belief into practice. I became aware of Carolyn and her pioneering work at Monte Nido years ago when I worked on an article about eating disorders and yoga. At the time I was excited to see a treatment center bold enough to offer yoga, not just as an elective but as an integral part of the healing process. And now that I've read *Yoga and Eating Disorders*, I'm thrilled to discover how her vision has expanded and how others are embracing yoga and incorporating it into their work. By sharing her expertise and offering a platform for other voices, Carolyn inspired a resource that provides practical advice for therapists and yoga teachers, as well as inspiration and hope for eating disordered sufferers. It's so heartening to see examples in these pages—from friends, colleagues and experts I admire so much—of how yoga has moved into populations it needs to serve. And the essays from young women who credit yoga with their own healing leave no doubt that it is serving them well.

For years I've worked with women who suffer from all kinds of body issues—women touched by cancer who feel their bodies have betrayed them; young girls who carry the scars and memories of abuse with shame and fear; older women who hate their wrinkled skin and can't abide what they see in the mirror. I used to believe that yoga would somehow make them better—stronger, more flexible, kinder to themselves, softer. I don't believe that anymore. I believe they already have everything they need to blossom and thrive—we all do.

What yoga does—with our help as teachers and therapists—is offer people a means to discover their own path toward wholeness and acceptance. In Chapter 13, Melody Moore, PhD, offers her students and clients an affirmation that speaks to that belief: *I am enough*. She doesn't say *I will be* or *I might be*, or *Maybe someday…* She says, *I AM*. A statement like that can empower women with eating disorders to move into their bodies safely, to lightly touch in for a moment and notice not only how, but what, they feel.

They may not be ready to dive too deeply, but a quick hello, a drive-by, can open the door to more exploration and, in time, profound healing. In order for that to happen, women need to connect with facilitators who practice yoga and embody the true teachings because, as Carolyn and the other experts within these pages so beautifully demonstrate, that's the only way yoga's gifts can light the way home.

Providence, Rhode Island
October, 2015

Linda Sparrowe is a long-time, widely-respected writer, editor, speaker and mentor in the holistic healing arena, with a special emphasis on women's health. As the former editor-in-chief of *Yoga International* magazine and managing editor of *Yoga Journal*, Linda has been instrumental in bringing the authentic voice of yoga to thousands of practitioners and teachers. Her latest book is *Yoga at Home* (Rizzoli, 2015). Learn more at lindasparrowe.com.

Introduction

The seeds for a book were planted in 1996 when I included yoga as part of the program at Monte Nido, my first residential center for eating disorders. Yoga had helped me after I recovered from anorexia and then developed an addiction to running. I thought (and hoped) yoga would be a good addition to the other treatment protocols we would offer eating disorder clients. I had no idea how profoundly yoga would contribute to the recovery of others, how integral yoga would become for all Monte Nido programs, and how valuable it would prove for other eating disorder professionals and sufferers around the world. The clients' reactions to yoga were beyond my expectations and began to foretell what was to come:

> Yoga gave me a healthy ritual to replace unhealthy ones. It provided me with a sense of community and connection. It forced me to challenge perfectionism because you can't be "good" at yoga; your body responds differently each day. If you push it, you hurt yourself and it gets you nowhere.

> Yoga provided me with healthy challenges that encouraged "stilling of the mind." Yoga encouraged gentleness and respect for my body.

> Yoga helped challenge me to stop comparing myself to others because everyone has such different strengths and weaknesses that have nothing to do with weight, talent or will power. Through yoga, I learned how connected my mind is to my body. For instance, my resistance to back bends encouraged me to think about my fear of opening up to people and being vulnerable, and I learned that balancing poses are difficult when my mind is distracted.

> In yoga class, I learned to meet myself in the authenticity and reality of the present moment. I learned to let myself unfold. Instead of finding myself pressured to do better or more, yoga encouraged listening to the nature of my humanity and respecting the signals my body, mind and soul offered. I met myself for the first time in as long as I could remember. What I had done in the past had not worked. Yoga gave me an alternative. I developed a belief in hope and the possibility to find

harmony within myself, apart from my surroundings. I found freedom
as I began to practice in my daily life all that I had found to be true on
the mat.

As the years progressed, I met countless other eating disorder professionals, yoga
teachers and sufferers having positive experiences using yoga as an aspect of
healing eating disorders. When my programs and clinical trainings expanded to
other states and countries, I also noticed a remarkable trend: a steadily increasing
number of eating disorder therapists and dietitians who were also certified yoga
teachers. As yoga practice and eating disorder recovery were finding their way to
each other, I felt compelled to explore, collect and communicate the growing
body of experience and knowledge. This book's seeds were now watered and
sprouting. I began communicating with people who I felt had important information to share, many of whom became contributing authors.

The people I have talked to, the teachers I have had and the authors in this
book study various types of yoga and have learned different aspects along the
way. However, all agree that the meaning of yoga is to unite or unify; in fact, the
word "yoga" comes from "yuj," a Sanskrit word meaning "to yoke" or to unite[1].

Yoga poses and philosophical teachings are designed to help human
beings unite mind with body, and reconnect them to their higher nature.
Yoga's numerous techniques are meant to facilitate increased awareness and
acceptance of what is and clarify what serves rather than hinders. The result
is less self-caused illusion and suffering, which leads to a state of inner harmony
often described as "spiritual." Thus, through yoga, one progressively
achieves greater unification of mind, body and spirit.

Yoga gave me a spiritual practice before I even knew it was happening.

If pondered for even a moment, it makes sense that this ancient philosophy
and practice might help someone with an eating disorder whose relationship
with mind, body and spirit is so tragically disrupted.

People with eating disorders are disconnected from, even at war with,
their bodies. Their minds are in a state of constant comparison. They are
judgmental of themselves and others, out of balance, caught in habitual
behavior patterns, and living in the past or future. As a yoga teacher said in
class just this morning, "Our bodies live mostly in the past and our minds in
the future; yoga helps us bring both into the present moment."

While yoga facilitates awareness, connection and unity of mind and body,
we do not claim that yoga *alone* can heal eating disorders. Instead, *Yoga*
and Eating Disorders: Ancient Healing for a Modern Illness demonstrates an
important role for yoga in an overall treatment strategy aimed at transforming
body dissatisfaction, disordered eating, addictive exercise, sabotaging thoughts
and self-destructive behaviors.

This book is about the combination of yoga and eating disorders and is
written by experienced eating disorder treatment professionals, researchers,

yoga teachers and yoga therapists. Some contributors are also recovered from their own eating disorder. Using personal stories, practical applications, teaching experiences, research studies and patient testimonials, these authors delineate why and how yoga works, while adding cautions about situations where human misuse and misinterpretation of yoga cause unintended and harmful outcomes. Collectively their work reveals that yoga offers benefits that other therapeutic modalities do not.

All suggestions, techniques and ideas in this book are meant to be used in conjunction with—not instead of—appropriate, standard treatment for eating disorders or other conditions.

As yoga's therapeutic benefits gain recognition, a growing number of physicians, nurses, psychologists, dietitians and other licensed health professionals are referring their patients to yoga. Several are becoming Registered Yoga Teachers, and using yoga in their practices. Meanwhile, some yoga teachers are taking additional training and calling themselves "Yoga Therapists." As of now it is difficult to differentiate the credentials, training and expertise between a yoga teacher and yoga therapist but efforts are being made by the International Association of Yoga Therapists (IAYT) and Yoga Alliance to establish standards.

It is incumbent upon all practitioners teaching yoga not to over step their training and skill set. For instance, yoga providers should not diagnose or treat health conditions unless they are trained and credentialed to do so.

If you are seeking yoga as a supplemental treatment for health conditions, it is imperative to carefully scrutinize the training and credentials of the yoga practitioner—and get approval from your primary health care provider(s) to participate.

On these pages readers will find descriptions of how yoga, when practiced appropriately, helps people become embodied beings and increases their awareness, acceptance and non-judgment.

This may seem like a simple concept, but it is very difficult to attain. Imagine for one minute that you are consciously in harmony with your body and mind,accepting *everything* for what it is, with openness and non-judgment. The scenario is hard to conceive, much less achieve, for anyone—and far more challenging for someone with an eating disorder whose mind and body are in battle.

When a person begins to practice yoga, balancing on one leg or doing even the simplest of backbends may seem impossible. Similarly, tasks that help someone recover from an eating disorder may also feel impossible at first. In both cases, with guidance, commitment and practice, what seemed difficult or impossible eventually comes naturally.

Yoga gave me hope that other things in my life could change because every time I practiced I noticed how things changed slightly and then eventually bigger changes would result.

In yoga and in recovery from an eating disorder, new skills are learned—first on the mat or in a therapy session. Then, they are incorporated into one's life as a whole, as a healthy and thriving way of being in the world.

Yoga and Eating Disorders is an attempt to explain something that can't really be explained, but has to be experienced over time to be understood. Whether a professional or sufferer, anyone interested in yoga or problems related to body image, eating, or exercise will find valuable resources in each chapter.

My hope is that *Yoga and Eating Disorders* will whet your appetite for greater knowledge, deeper understanding and the desire for personal exploration.

Namaste,
Carolyn Costin MA, MEd, MFT
February 4, 2016
Malibu, California

Please visit our website, www.YogaAndEatingDisorders.com, *for links to illustrations and videos which demonstrate the poses (asanas) mentioned in this book. The site also has links to articles and other resources on the relationship between yoga and eating disorders.*

Note

1 Merriam-Webster Digital Dictionary; www.merriam-webster.com/dictionary/yoga (retrieved 7/14/2015).

Part 1

Why and How Yoga Helps Heal Eating Disorders

1 Yoga: A Healing Journey, from Personal to Professional

Carolyn Costin

People with eating disorders have become disconnected from their true selves and lost their way. Every eating disorder client who walks through my door seeking help has a healthy soul self deep inside, but a disordered self has taken over and is running the show.

Eating disorders develop due to a combination of risk factors such as gender, genetic vulnerability, cultural weight and shape pressures and other psychological variables (e.g., anxiety or a trauma history). On a deeper level, there is profound disconnection.

These clients are disconnected from their body. They stop listening, paying attention to and responding to their body's signals. They stop appreciating and caring for their body altogether. What may have seemed like caring in the beginning, "I want to be trim," or "I need to lose weight to get healthy," becomes something entirely different and takes on a life of its own.

At 79 pounds, a girl with anorexia is no longer restricting food to be healthy or trim, but because her brain simply tells her to. She is lost, not only disconnected from her body, but from her own mind, which has been hijacked. Her way of relating to her body and to food has been rewired in her brain and new circuits have created a pattern she can't escape. Luckily, we can retrain the mind to change the brain. We can also help her connect her body, mind and soul.

When disconnected from soul, both body and mind run amok. The mind or ego, which thrives on personal identity and achievement, is attached to things like grades, status, appearance and control.

Untethered to soul and the truth of what *really* matters, things of the ego take on undue importance but can never be fully satisfying. All kinds of maladies such as depression, anxiety, addictions and eating disorders result. How do we heal such disconnection?

The Bemba people of Zambia believe that every human being comes into the world as valuable. Everyone is eager to love and have peace, connection and happiness. However, sometimes, in the pursuit of these things, people make mistakes. The Bemba see those mistakes as a cry for help.

If you are a member of the tribe and have done something wrong or harmful the Bemba take you to the center of the village for a ritual called

Shikoba Nabajyotisaikia. For two days, they tell you all the good things you've done. The tribe believes you made a mistake and it is their responsibility to lift you up and reconnect you with your true nature; to remind you, until you can remember, the full truth from which you are temporarily disconnected[1].

How can we help those with eating disorders remember the full truth and reconnect to their true nature? Eradicating the symptoms of an eating disorder is a challenging task; even harder is healing on a deeper level. Yoga can help with both.

Yoga and meditation author Michael Singer writes: "The very essence of spirituality is represented by the question 'Who are you that is lost and trying to build a concept of yourself in order to be found?'"[2]

Yoga is an ancient philosophy and practice in existence since as early as 300 BCE. If one goes back far enough there are hundreds, maybe thousands, of yoga poses and various teachings. Yoga philosophy and practices are designed as a means of transcending the idea that "I am my body." (Hence one can find early yoga references denigrating the body.)

Originally handed down only orally, a man or several men called "Patanjali" compiled various yogic teachings and summarized the ancient art and science of yoga somewhere between 400 BCE and 200 AD. This work, known as the *Yoga Sutras*, includes the "Eight Fold Path" or "Eight Limbs of Yoga," and has been translated countless times.[3] Yoga poses or postures, called Asanas, are the third limb and thus only one part of a rich overall yoga philosophy and practice.

The Yoga Sutras are designed to help with understanding the nature and function of the mind and consciousness. They provide techniques and practices geared to cease the rampant activity of the mind, allowing for connection to a deeper awareness, to one's true self and to everything else in the universe. This alone can reduce needless self-caused pain and suffering. It is thought that consistent practice brings self-realization and allows one to transcend the self and rest in his or her own true divine spirit or nature.[4]

When I learned what yoga really is, I was already familiar with many of the concepts and ideas from my exploration of Buddhist teachings. Like Buddhism, yoga is a philosophy of living and self-realization, not a faith based practice. Neither require belief in anything other-worldly, thus people of any religion, or none, can practice. I was already incorporating Buddhist ideas in my work with eating disorder clients, such as teaching the difference between their ego/mind and their core essence or soul self.

Yoga fit right in as a way to enhance and physically concretize what I was trying to do: help clients realize that the eating disorder self is ego/mind out of control. Help them understand that they are not their eating disorder self. Help them separate from it and re-connect with their true nature or soul. Once connected to soul, things like weight get into proper perspective, where a number on a scale is no longer a matter of consequence.

My introduction to yoga was an accident and came about when I decided to try it as a replacement form of exercise. Years earlier I had recovered from anorexia nervosa but my driven, tenacious temperament had turned my attention toward running and created an internal obligation to do so. Multiple stress fractures were now preventing me from putting on my Nikes and heading for the hills, and I was desperate for an alternative.

Fifteen minutes into my first yoga class, I was distraught and tears began to form. "This is not exercise," I thought. "I will never be able to stay in shape doing this." Though I cried, things about the class intrigued me, so I continued to go.

It didn't take long before I realized that my body was actually getting stronger in new and interesting ways, but far more was also taking place. For the first time in a long time, I was listening to my body, paying attention to how it moved and felt, noticing how my breath could help or hinder me. Through yoga I developed a new kind of respect for my body, improving it with patience rather than pushing and encouragement rather than the "no pain, no gain" attitude I had been functioning under for many years.

Throughout the classes, my yoga teachers wove concepts that I already knew and valued, such as mindful awareness, acceptance verses resistance, and self-compassion. Practicing these concepts through movement and mind/body awareness helped me physically embody them, making them more tangible. I learned that "Asana" was derived from a Sanskrit word meaning "seated," because practicing the postures or poses was supposed to help one sit in meditation. Patanjali describes asana as "a comfortable, steady pose." I found this intriguing because meditation had always been hard for me but yoga was helping me slow down, pay attention internally, and become aware of my awareness, which was the closest I had ever been to what I understood meditation to be.

My knowledge of the history of yoga barely scratches the surface. I am not adept at any particular form of yoga. I don't call myself a devotee of any kind of yogic philosophy. What I know is that yoga, as a practice and philosophy, helped me embody what I already cognitively understood was true. It helped me live in my body with awareness, respect, non-judgment, harmony and honor. It enhanced my ability to be still, go inside, maintain balance, avoid comparison and be in the moment, yet not totally disconnected from the past or future. Practicing yoga taught me to accept where I was while, at the same time, guiding me to improve.

If yoga did all this for me, how could it not be beneficial for my clients? I began recommending yoga to certain clients in my private practice. At the hospital eating disorder unit, where I served as clinical director, I lobbied to hire a yoga teacher for the patients. I was denied. Then, in 1996, I decided to open my own program, Monte Nido, the first residential eating disorder facility licensed in a home setting. I asked my yoga teacher, Lauren Peterson,[5] to provide yoga philosophy and practice as part of our services.

A few reactions were surprising, for example: "I'm not sure I can come to Monte Nido because yoga might be against my religion." Some clients thought they would have to meditate, do headstands or put their feet behind their head. Several were disappointed that yoga was in place of "real" exercise. Even though the program included walking and fitness training with weights, they wanted to run; they wanted treadmills and stair stepping machines.

Though yoga is now far better understood, and is often included in treatment settings, resistance still persists in some clients and professionals. However, those who experience it learn that yoga is not what they thought and, although an excellent form of physical exercise, it offers far more than they ever expected.

As one client explains:

> *When I attended the first yoga class at Monte Nido I thought at least it would be better than sitting in group.*
>
> *When the teacher started by having us sit on the floor, I thought I would lose it. As she spoke about the theme of the class, I started paying attention. She was talking about the feeling of being "centered" and asked us if we had a concept of what that was like. She asked us to sit in a way that we felt centered on the mat and to notice how it feels. Then she got us to stand up, lean to the left and notice the non-centered feeling, then ever so gently try to find "center" in that position. She helped us go from center to off center in various poses, feeling "off" until finding our center of gravity. I noticed my body working to be centered and me paying attention to it and helping it. I noticed how it felt to be able to find my center, to get grounded, even when at first it seemed out of my reach.*
>
> *At the end of the class the teacher asked us to think about where we feel centered in our lives. She asked what throws us off center and if and how we listen to what our body tells us. She asked us to see if, during the next week, we could gently guide ourselves back to center when we get pulled off. I was astonished. I felt the teacher was talking to me. I enjoyed moving in the poses and working at doing them "correctly" but I had been moved in another way. To this day, in all areas of my life, I use the centering lessons and all the lessons I learned and continue to learn in yoga.*

How Yoga Transforms Exercise

Fifteen years of treating eating disorders prior to opening Monte Nido taught me the importance of incorporating healthy exercise. Taking away all exercise, as was the general practice, did not work. In private practice a no exercise rule is almost impossible to enforce. When enforced under 24-hour care, clients go right back to unhealthy exercise habits after discharging. Monte Nido has a gym, exercise equipment and a fitness trainer, but it is yoga that profoundly transforms our clients' approach to exercise in a new and healthy way. Of course, many clients are initially interested in yoga because it purports to provide some kind of exercise. Yet, whatever clients come in the front door expecting, yoga provides a back door into teaching them much more:

> *Yoga was the first time I could do exercise without trying to calculate calories burned. At first I hated it because I thought it wouldn't do anything, then I saw my body change. I saw that where in the beginning I could hardly touch my shins, I soon could touch my toes. I realized that with patience I developed the capability of doing the splits where I had thought it would never happen. Yoga taught me to accept and be where I am with my body. I found myself for the first time being really interested in how my body felt, not how it looked. I could have never ever imagined that.*

Yoga teaches us how to be "in" our body, use our body, and take care of our body with understanding, awareness and acceptance.

Is Yoga Appropriate and Safe For Use With Clients Who Have Eating Disorders?

I believe yoga can help all eating disorder clients. However, some professionals wonder: "Are you sure the clients should be exercising?" "How many calories are they burning?" "Should people with anorexia even do yoga?" "Is it medically safe?"

These questions indicate a misunderstanding of yoga. "Doing yoga" can mean practicing poses, doing breathing exercises, speaking the truth without judgment or meditating. Treatment providers should be sure clients are medically cleared to practice poses.[6] However, yoga is about working at one's own level and body limitations. This means all clients should be able to do something appropriate for their body and their circumstances.

In terms of calorie burning, clients will obviously burn more calories doing yoga poses than sitting in a therapy session or group. There are severely emaciated clients who should not be doing active yoga poses. In treatment, clients who do not finish a meal or purge should be excused from engaging in an asana practice. All the above said, most yoga asana classes are not excessively vigorous and burn fewer calories than one might expect.

A study of Hatha yoga found that the highest energy expenditure reached (during the most challenging poses) was 3.02 kcal per minute for the average female. Even if the entire class was all high intensity, the calories burned in 60 minutes would come to about 181kcal.[7] Few yoga classes consist entirely of high intensity poses. Even Hot Yoga classes such as Bikram styles don't burn as much as many people think. Colorado State University professor Brian Tracy tested the metabolic rate of 11 females and eight males, ages 18 to 40, during a 90-minute Bikram Yoga session. He found that the women burned an average of 330 calories and men 460.[8] Nevertheless, I don't recommend vigorous classes with little to no yoga philosophy for clients with eating disorders. (This book provides readers with knowledge to make informed decisions about yoga practices to recommend or participate in.)

Yoga *can* decrease eating disorder symptoms while not decreasing BMI. In a study of eating disorder clients, ages 11 through 21, the control group received "standard care" (physician and dietitian visits), while the test group received standard care along with individualized yoga. The yoga group demonstrated greater decreases in eating disorder symptoms a month after their treatment, while the control group showed some initial decline but then returned to baseline levels.[9] Food preoccupation dropped significantly after all yoga sessions. Both groups maintained BMI levels and experienced decreased anxiety and depression over time. The researchers conclude: "Results suggest individualized yoga therapy holds promise as adjunctive therapy to standard [eating disorders] care."[10]

Yoga Lessons Applied to Recovery and Life

Learning a concept through yoga makes it easier to see how the same principle applies elsewhere. Yoga helps instill concepts and beliefs that apply to the client's treatment and overall life. For example, at the end of most yoga classes, clients are asked to practice savasana, also known as corpse pose, where the person lies down on the mat, face up, eyes closed, just quietly being. People with eating disorders are often restless, anxious and feel obligated to be "doing," so savasana is one of the hardest poses for them. It may take a while for some clients to even close their eyes.

How clients handle savasana is usually an indicator of how they are doing in other areas of treatment and life. When better at savasana, clients are usually better at focusing or soothing themselves in general. Savasana specifically and yoga in general helps quiet a chattering mind and allows for acceptance of simply being in the moment. This is a formidable task for anyone, but especially for people with the constant banter of an eating disorder mind.

Mind/Body Connection:

Neuroscience has made the importance of the mind/body connection abundantly clear, particularly in relationship to healing. Neuroplasticity shows that the mind and body are important partners. When working together our mind/body team can heal our brains and even help people recover faculties lost as a result of traumatic brain injuries, strokes, or illnesses like Parkinson's.[11]

What we are learning about mindfulness practices, eating disorders and the brain suggests that over the next several years, mind/body techniques will show increasing efficacy in treating eating disorders. Psychiatrist and

UCLA Medical School professor Dan Siegel is the pioneer of Interpersonal neurobiology which encompasses the way our mind, brain and body work to create a sense of who we are. Siegel is among many to suggest that eating disorders are disorders of self-awareness.[12]

Yoga is one of the easiest ways to facilitate and develop mind/body awareness and connection. For example, when practicing yoga one learns that certain body postures are related to certain moods, that accomplishing a head stand requires letting go of one's preconceived ideas, and that you can subtly correct a posture without coming out of the pose if you stay in the present with mind/body awareness. Furthermore, the mind/body connection developed on the mat helps clients develop the same skill off it.

> *Through yoga, I learned how connected my mind is to my body. I learned that balancing poses are difficult when my mind is distracted. This helped me pay attention to how and when I get distracted in my life.*

> *My resistance to back bends and how they initially made me feel unsafe encouraged me to think about my fear of opening up to people and being vulnerable.*

> *Yoga re-connected my mind and body into a friendship that had been destroyed by my eating disorder. This friendship stays together off the mat and into the larger world every day of my life.*

Accepting and Non-Comparing

Yoga offers reminders of the need to accept where you are even while trying to change. In yoga you must work with your own body and at your own pace. To try to perform poses like someone else will not work. You have to do what is right for your body, learn your own strengths and weaknesses, discover how far to push and when to let go.

> *Yoga helped challenge me to stop comparing myself to others. Not being able to do a hip opener has nothing to do with being better than somebody else. Everyone has such different strengths and weaknesses that have nothing to do with weight, talent, will power or worthiness.*

Through yoga we get constant feedback that comparing ourselves to others on or off the mat can undermine and derail our own process.

The Need for Balance and "Doing the Harder Thing"

In yoga you have to learn *not* to stick to poses you like or are easy for you. You have to also practice doing what is harder, otherwise you get strong in some areas while remaining weak in others and your overall progress will be affected.

"Doing the harder thing" does not mean to push beyond safety, or ignore all signals and do something anyway. It means trying things that seem hard or challenging while paying attention to your body and working with it. It means backing off when you need to, rather than avoiding something because you are not good at it or it seems "too hard" to even attempt.

When I began practicing yoga I was very flexible and found it easy to do backbends, often choosing them over other poses. Some students and teachers impressed by my flexibility encouraged me to try increasingly advanced versions such as scorpion pose. Rather than equally practicing poses to strengthen my stomach and arms such as navanasa (boat pose), essentially a sit up, or chattarungas (pushups), I over-focused on accomplishing scorpion. Soon my ability to achieve an advanced flexibility pose exceeded my strength to execute it safely. My body and skills were seriously out of balance and I sustained injuries. Yoga taught me in a concrete way that to achieve balance and to progress I had to stop choosing things that I liked, were easier, or impressed others. I had to practice doing the harder things.

I incorporate "doing the harder thing" off the mat and into eating disorder recovery by guiding clients to not always choose foods they consider safe, thus easier to eat, such as salad or grilled chicken. In order to strengthen their healthy self, clients need to try "scary" foods that are harder to eat, like pizza. It's not that eating pizza is critical for recovery, but doing the harder thing builds the *strength* and *flexibility* to eat scary foods without feeling guilt, shame, or the need to binge, purge and/or restrict. Whether practicing a variety of poses or choosing a variety of foods, balance is key. Practicing yoga helps clients embrace the need for balance and embody doing the harder thing, serving up reminders to apply this lesson in all areas of life.

Combining Behaviors with Meaning to Facilitate Lasting Change

Major transformation through yoga does not take place simply by doing poses. Asanas are nothing but body movements unless one also learns and incorporates yoga's philosophical principles. The Eight Limbs of yoga include Yoga's Yamas, or tenets of moral conduct; Niyamas, ethical and spiritual observances; and the Koshas, or the subtle layers of our being. All of these underlie an informed yoga practice and are uncanny in their beneficial use in eating disorder recovery.[13] These concepts include accepting the present moment and one's experience; being truthful to one's feelings, thoughts, words, and actions; balance; the importance of one's breath; compassion for self and others; non-reliance on external validation, and connection to true self.

These are all useful concepts for those with eating disorders. In fact, the numerous concepts and principles involved in a fully rounded yoga practice are useful for healing, not just from an eating disorder, but from any disorder or affliction. It is the combination of practicing the asanas along with the meaning and purpose behind them that brings about transformative, lasting change from yoga.

Taking this concept off the mat can help both clinicians and clients understand why distinct eating disorder recovery skills (such as writing a behavior chain analysis, journaling before a binge, or doing a Cognitive Behavioral Therapy exercise) are unlikely, in isolation, to lead to lasting transformation. Recovery behaviors need to be connected to one another and to a deeper meaning and purpose that is understood and "felt." There is a "how" to recovery but there is also a "why." Yoga philosophy is a guide to help with both. When clients can weave their recovery tasks and behavioral skills together, and to the deeper purpose of connection with their true essence or soul self, it enhances their motivation and ability to continue "practicing recovery" until a new healthy, soul centered way of relating to food and one's body becomes a natural way of life and then they are Recovered.

Like Mindedness, Relationships, and Community

Many clients say that the treatment community and the relationships formed are a large part of what they find helpful to their recovery. Upon leaving treatment clients essentially lose this "community." A yoga practice can give clients a ready-made community and place to belong. All they have to do is find a yoga class or others doing yoga. Clients often find a yoga studio where they continue to practice yoga *and* discover a group of like-minded individuals. Some people find connection or comfort simply going in and out of the community when taking classes while others have met new friends, been introduced to various reading materials and teachings, discovered useful workshops or retreats and even met lifelong partners.

Final Thoughts

This chapter is a small summary of an expedition I am still on. Those of us combining yoga and the treatment of eating disorders are all on a journey of discovery. So far, the good I have seen come from yoga far outweighs any of the concerns I had for using it with the eating disorder population. I personally tried yoga and it helped. Then I offered yoga to the clients at Monte Nido as an experiment, and it also helped, beyond my wildest dreams. I detail observations and lessons from my experience in my later chapter, Opening the Door to Yoga in Treatment.

I have had many great teachers, including my clients and every contributor to this book. All of us continue to learn more about ourselves and the various ways in which yoga works, or doesn't work and why. I feel an enormous amount of gratitude for having been able to introduce yoga, and my experience using it with eating disorders, to thousands of clients and clinicians over the years.

Though, in this chapter, I only briefly touch on the details of my own personal to professional journey with yoga, the rest of this book fills in gaps, answers questions and discusses ideas that readers might already have contemplated thus far. It is a great pleasure to have you with us on this journey.

Namaste.

Notes

1 See: www.africanamerica.org/topic/shikoba-nabajyotisaikia-is-this-the-answer. (Retrieved 7/13/2015.)

2 Singer, Michael A. *The Untethered Soul: The Journey beyond Yourself* (Oakland, CA: New Harbinger, 2007).

3 Whicher, Ian. *The Integrity of the Yoga Darsana: A Reconsideration of the Classical Yoga* (Albany, NY: State University of New York Press, 1999), p. 49.

4 Iyengar, B.K.S. *Light on the Yoga Sutras of Patanjali* (London, UK: Thorsons, 2002).

5 See Lauren's perspective in chapter 5.

6 See later chapters by Diers, Hussa Farrell and Mott.

7 Ray, U.S., Pathak A. and Tomer, O.S. (2011) "Hatha yoga practices: Energy expenditure, respiratory changes and intensity of exercise" in *Evidenced Based Complementary Alternative Medicine Volume 2011*. Article ID: 241294.

8 Presentation by Brian Tracy at the American Conference of Sports Medicine's 2014 national meeting in Orlando, Florida.

9 Carei, T.R., Fyfe-Johnson, A.L., Breuner, C.C., and Marshall, M.A. (2010) "Randomized controlled clinical trial of yoga in the treatment of eating disorders" in *Journal of Adolescent Health*, 46(4): 346–351.

10 *Ibid.*

11 Doidge, Norman. *The Brain's Way of Healing: Remarkable Discoveries and Recoveries from the Frontiers of Neuroplasticity* (New York: Viking, 2015).

12 Siegel, Daniel J. *The Mindful Therapist: A Clinician's Guide to Mindsight and Neural Integration* (New York: W.W. Norton, 2010), p. 41.

13 See Sobara Mora's chapter on Yamas and Niyamas.

2 Yamas and Niyamas on the Journey to Recovery from Eating Disorders

Maria Sorbara Mora

Yoga is more than a physical practice of body postures; it is a harmonizing system of development for the body, mind and spirit. I believe yoga can facilitate treatment for eating disorders, help sustain the recovery process, and inspire sacred meaning in life. As a Registered Dietitian and eating disorder specialist for many years I was unsatisfied with what our field had to offer those who were struggling. When I began practicing yoga I found not only my own life change but I also found my approach to counseling changed as well. I began using the word "healing" instead of recovery or treatment. The philosophy yoga offered, integration of body and soul, resonated with me on a deep level.

After several years of suggesting to my patients that they consider yoga as a practice for healing, I realized what was missing from my own work. I became certified from a mind-body yoga therapy called Phoenix Rising Yoga Therapy[1] and went on to become the founder of Body Connection, the first yoga studio devoted to the healing of those with eating disorders. In this chapter I examine two valuable aspects of yoga philosophy, the Yamas and Niyamas. The Yamas, tenets of moral conduct, and the Niyamas, ethical and spiritual observances, underlie an informed yoga practice and are beneficial principles for use in eating disorder recovery.

The practice of yoga makes the body strong and flexible, improving the function of respiratory, circulatory, digestive, and hormonal systems. It also brings about emotional stability and clarity of mind. The recovery journey requires the same. When recovered from an eating disorder, food, eating and one's body are joyful, comforting elements of living.

The understanding and practice of yoga embrace connection to something greater than ourselves. In the Yoga Sutras, Patanjali identified the Eightfold Path or the Eight Limbs of Yoga, which lead toward the goal of self-realization:[2]

Yamas: Tenets of moral conduct which include widely treasured human characteristics known for centuries as key to living one's life in freedom.

Niyamas: Observances that foster the ethical and spiritual aspects of the self.

Asanas: Postures that keep the body strong, flexible and relaxed, while strengthening the nervous system and refining inner perception.

Pranayama: The practice of breathing to foster movement of one's life force.

Pratyahara: Drawing one's attention toward silence through withdrawal of the senses from external objects.

Dharana: Focused concentration holds the mind to one thought or object.

Dhyana: Meditation aims for sustaining awareness of the Divine under all conditions.

Samadhi: The super-conscious experience of oneness of the soul with the Cosmic Spirit, and the return of the mind into original silence.

All eight limbs are equally important but most westerners are familiar only with the third limb, Asanas, or the yoga postures. The first two limbs, Yamas and Niyamas, teach us how to be compassionate, generous, honest and peaceful. These teachings show us that the techniques of yoga are not goals in themselves, but vehicles for getting to the essence of who we are.

When you become familiar with the Yamas and Niyamas, you can see how practicing them deepens our relationship to our true self and to other people. I will describe each Yama and Niyama and then explain their relevance from the perspective of a person in treatment and recovery *as well as* from the perspective of family members, loved ones, clinicians, treatment providers and others.[3]

Yamas

In yoga, Yamas are tenets of moral conduct that include widely treasured human characteristics known for centuries as keys to living one's life in freedom. The five Yama principles are: Ahimsa, Satya, Asteya, Brahmacharya and Aparigraha.

Ahimsa: Non-Violence

Ahimsa is the practice of abstaining from being "violent" or hurtful in one's thoughts, words, feelings, or actions. Ahimsa is the foundation of the other Yamas because it is the stance of "right relationships." Practicing Ahimsa, we learn to have compassion and kindness for others and for ourselves.[4]

For People with Eating Disorders

Those with eating disorders often are generous towards others but lack self-compassion. Forced starvation, chaotic bingeing, purging, draining over-exercise, numbing overeating and other eating disorder behaviors can be seen as forms of self-inflicted violence. When asked if they would recommend or force anyone else to engage in these behaviors, individuals with eating disorders generally seem appalled at the idea.

Practicing Ahimsa involves following advice one would give others; thus replacing negative, self-violating thoughts and symptoms with more compassionate and healthy alternatives. For example, one of my patients has learned that: "When I 'feel fat' or consider myself 'unworthy,' I remind myself not to go into the 'bad neighborhoods' of my head. Instead, I work on staying in the 'safer' neighborhoods."

Ahimsa's emphasis on non-violence often moves people to choose vegetarianism or veganism, in order to reduce violence against animals. However, people with eating disorders may hide behind the ethical aspects of vegetarianism to justify and protect their eating behavior. Therefore, therapists and dietitians should explore a patient's reasons for choosing or not choosing to eat certain foods in order to help them see whether the choice is coming from a place of Ahimsa, or is symptomatic of the eating disorder.

Since many patients walk in the door as staunch vegans or vegetarians, it is important to approach this topic in a way that demonstrates respect for their current food choices, while also inviting them to listen to and honor their body's requirements. These individuals need to be educated, challenged, and encouraged to examine the relationship between their choice to abstain from meat and/or animal products and their body's wants and needs.

It helps to explain how Ahimsa requires us to first extend non-violence inwards to support our own life functions. We cannot practice non-violence towards others without demonstrating real compassion for ourselves. With this understanding, individuals with eating disorders may come to view their behaviors from a different light and may begin to make choices that show a greater regard for their body's needs—even if that means eating meat.

We see Ahimsa reality all around us; the mother bird must feed herself before she feeds her baby birds, and, in an airline emergency, we must don our own masks before helping our children with theirs. Yoga acknowledges the tremendous value of practicing Ahimsa first towards our self, body, thoughts, feelings, actions and experiences before extending it towards others.

Ahimsa requires learning to respect the body and its boundaries. This means honoring hunger and fullness cues, while maintaining a healthy relationship to food and exercise. Ahimsa is a manifestation of recovery.

For Providers and Loved Ones

Ahimsa is about self-care and self-compassion. Effectively supporting a person through treatment and recovery requires a tremendous amount of endurance. Caregivers and clinicians share the complex task of providing support while maintaining their own strength and avoiding over-involvement and burnout. Incorporating a regular self-care practice such as seeking outside counseling for oneself and establishing healthy boundaries can prevent exhaustion while also maintaining the effectiveness of the support provided. Furthermore, regular monitoring of one's own feelings and needs (and demonstrating compassion for those feelings and needs) allows caregivers and clinicians to ascertain risk of burnout and help them remain invested in the treatment process.

Satya: Truthfulness

Satya is based on the understanding that honest communication and action is the foundation of all healthy relationships while deception, exaggeration and dishonesty are harmful to everyone involved. Satya is intimately connected with ahimsa because it builds on the premise that lying and dishonesty are forms of violence. Practicing Satya means being truthful to one's feelings, thoughts, words and actions.

> *Recovery is like lifting a fog and being able to see things as they actually are.*
> A recovered patient

For People with Eating Disorders

An eating disorder stifles the truth, keeping the person from the essence of who they are and causing them to deny or lie about what they think and feel. Dishonesty and distortion are frequently part of the presentation. Body image distortion, a hallmark symptom for many eating disorders, is a prime example. The person's brain is unable to perceive his or her own body accurately and believes the distorted or "untrue" perceptions. Irrational or distorted thoughts, such as, "I'm worthless" or "I'm not good enough," and irrational thinking, such as "If I eat fat, I will get fat" or "Bingeing on ice cream will make things better," dominate the person's thinking and need to be challenged.

Lying and denial are often entrenched patterns in people with eating disorders. They may lie about what or how much they ate or if they engaged in any compensatory behaviors such as purging or over-exercise. They may deny the problem altogether or how bad their problem is: "Everyone eats too much sometimes," "Why are you so obsessed with my weight?" or "I'm not sick; I still get my period." They might engage in their behaviors while denying their basic needs, covering them up or numbing them. Some may even refuse to drink water, resist sleep, and not allow themselves to rest when sick.

Shedding denial is difficult because it means letting go of stories and beliefs that caused or were perpetuated by the eating disorder and eventually became entrenched in the person's brain. Years of disordered eating behaviors reinforce the fiction that the person is inherently flawed and unlovable.

Recovery involves Satya, the process of becoming honest with oneself and others. Satya teaches us to peel away layers of denial and distorted belief, leaving irrational thinking behind.

Practicing Satya we work to be aware of false perceptions and choose not to believe we are our old stories. Satya brings people back to their truth and allows deeper connection to themselves and others.

As individuals nourish their bodies and manage symptoms, they also regain the ability to see themselves more accurately. One of my yoga therapy clients recently told me, "I have been able to realize that I am not broken, and that I am worthy of loving relationships." For this patient, recovery challenged her to question the "old" and untrue stories she learned so well.

The eating disorder is paradoxical in that it can function as both an expression and denial of needs. Critically important is the power of Satya, or truth telling, to help someone reclaim her or his voice and express needs.

When recovered from eating disorders, individuals use their voice to honestly express their feelings, wants, needs and desires. When practicing Satya, one communicates and acts in accordance with one's true needs, including those of the body. Living in Satya, we can open ourselves up to the world and consider our heart's true desire and destiny.

For Providers and Loved Ones

It is important to think, speak and act with honesty when engaging with ourselves and those we care about. Of course, this is easier said than done.

Practicing Satya means not colluding with the struggling individual's eating disorder self. When we notice denial in our patients, clients, students, or loved ones we need to come to them as an honest and compassionate mirror. We cannot help the person if we appease the disorder's denial. Instead, we must gently and consistently confront the eating disorder and call out for truth.

Health care professionals often feel apprehensive about confronting patients about their eating disorders, fearing the person will become upset, reject further care, and continue to jeopardize their health. Most health care professionals are not trained or well-versed in the treatment of eating disorders, yet they are often the first providers to recognize the symptoms and encounter the denial that so frequently accompanies the disorder.

Practicing Satya should not involve being mean, accusatory, or judgmental. Aggressively confronting people with judgment or negative energy won't work. Satya means firmly and compassionately speaking the truth with the patient and calmly pointing out the facts and the concern without any judgment or negativity.

For example, "You are underweight, your heartbeat is irregular, and you report feeling dizzy when you go from sitting to standing. These symptoms make me seriously concerned about your health."

If the patient retreats into denial, the provider can gently lead him or her back to the facts and suggest professional help from a specialist. Being gentle and kind but firm in telling the truth can facilitate huge transformations.

Although not easy, speaking the truth without judgment in the presence of entrenched, clever and illogical denial is necessary to reach someone struggling with an eating disorder, even when we encounter anger and retaliation.

Satya helps us recognize that:

- The retaliation is not about us and what we said (it's the disorder's reaction to being "called out" and confronted).
- Anger is common and can serve a purpose (a patient's anger signals that, at least on some level, there are feelings and engagement).
- The truth is a real consequence, and consequences undermine denial. On the other hand, attempts to manipulate or deny the denial merely prolong it.

Satya goes beyond overcoming denial or lying and becomes a constant practice of awareness and honesty about one's thoughts and behaviors. Through Satya individuals are constantly offered opportunities for growth and transformation.

Like recovery, Satya does not require us to be perfect. However, it does mean being honest about our own issues.

Many eating disorder clinicians are drawn to the work, at least in part, by their own personal experiences. It is also common for some of our patients' family members to struggle with disordered eating, too.

Loved ones and providers should not avoid an honest review of their own relationships and behaviors in regards to food and our bodies. No matter who we are—a passionate clinician, a soulful yoga teacher, or a concerned family member—we too need to practice Satya and assess how honest we are with ourselves regarding our own body image and eating.

Satya guides us in using our experiences to inform our work and/or responses to the disorder and how it develops. For instance, recovery means the person is on a Satya path, where he or she neutrally assesses the facts and chooses to be honest with self and others. The same holds true for providers and family.

Satya includes being honest about how one is reacting to another person's eating disorder. An eating disorder affects more than just the person with the disorder and can either directly or indirectly cause harm to anyone in the vicinity. All involved must ask, "Can I neutrally assess and identify the facts? Can I express my feelings, considering how angry, afraid, frustrated, and impotent I feel in the presence of the eating disorder?"

It can be quite disturbing and painful to watch a family member with their own eating issues focus solely on the patient's disorder and not deal with their own. Conversely, it can be enormously healing to witness a parent disclose that he or she too is struggling. In this case, the practice of Satya, or honesty, validates what the client and family likely sensed all along and ultimately invites a greater degree of healing

Asteya: Non-Stealing

In yoga philosophy, stealing occurs when one perceives the world as lacking abundance and fears there is not enough of something to satisfy needs and desires. Sadly, our marketing-driven culture continuously reinforces the idea that we are not enough, we do not have enough, and that achieving a better life requires the accumulation of external objects, beauty and affirmations. When we feel we are "not enough" we seek outside sources to feed or fill ourselves, causing the tendency to grasp for (and sometimes even steal) what is not rightfully ours. Outright theft is not good behavior by anyone's standards, but the issue goes deeper. Whether or not one literally steals things, the underlying problem is the cycle of looking for external sources of satisfaction and abundance. Living in that cycle, we fall further away from the ability to appreciate the abundance that already exists within us.

For People with Eating Disorders

People with eating disorders commonly report feeling like they are "not enough" or think they will be happier and more satisfied, once they achieve a certain goal (such as a number on the scale). Of course, reaching those goals is never enough. A person who binges on food will never be satisfied by a binge, and someone who restricts food will never lose enough weight to create the desired meaning and wholeness. They are ultimately attempting to find happiness and satisfaction where it can't be found.

Their symptoms can represent:

- A search for external validation: "When I'm thin enough, people will love me."
- A way of coping with not measuring up: "I can't get what I want, so I might as well binge."
- A way to manage a lack of self-worth: "When I binge and purge, I numb myself from all other feelings."

People with eating disorders steal food, laxatives, or other objects in the service of their eating disorder. These behaviors usually bring a lot of guilt, humiliation and shame to people with eating disorders and should be addressed with discernment and empathy. One method to interrupt this pattern and address the root of the problem is through understanding and practicing Asteya. Asteya helps nourish and develop inner resources instead of continuing to look outward.

Answering questions like "What has my eating disorder stolen from me?" and "How does my eating disorder keep me from enjoying the things I have?" helps clients discover how the eating disorder actually *robs them* of things they need or desire, rather than providing them.

In response to one of these questions, a client of mine recently reflected on how her drive for thinness and fear of building bulk kept her from doing any strengthening exercises and ultimately prevented her from having a strong body.

For Providers and Loved Ones

Practicing Asteya invites loved ones to ask questions such as: What has the eating disorder stolen from me or my family? How does the eating disorder keep my family and me from enjoying what we have? For many families, it is easy to recognize the ways in which the eating disorder robs all members of the family of fun, attention, and quality time. Here are a few ideas of how family members can practice Asteya:

- Make intentional, quality, one-on-one time devoted to each member of the family as an individual.
- Engage in your own self-care; paradoxically self-care is an excellent way to challenge the eating disorder.
- Remind yourself that right behind the façade of the eating disorder is the authentic person you love and miss. Your loved one is not an eating disorder.

For providers, the practice of Asteya means examining what we lack and how that may show up in the therapeutic relationship. We must ask ourselves if we are truly being with our clients in their journey or are we focusing too much on the outcome? Are we "stealing" their recovery or lack of progress by taking undue responsibility for it? It can be easy to take undue credit for successes and failures with clients. Certainly, we are part of the process, but as practitioners, we must not take away from their process and we must remind them of their capacity and inner wisdom for self-healing. In this way, we are practicing the essence of Asteya by realizing we all have enough and are enough.

Brahmacharya: Non-excess

In simple terms, Brahmacharya translates into *balance* of energy or life force—what yogis call "prana."

In a culture that thrives on intensity ("no pain, no gain" and "work hard, play hard"), being out of balance is not just a common malady; it is idealized. We impulsively sleep too little, work too hard, spend too much, and are regularly praised for these behaviors. We abuse alcohol, drugs, coffee, exercise, sex, etc. in order to fill unmet needs, only to be pulled further out of balance by the consequences of these behaviors (i.e. fatigue, hangovers and irritability).

The practice of Brahmacharya teaches us how to manage our impulses and consciously choose how and when to move energy so that our prana or life force doesn't become excessive in one way or another. Brahmacharya thus creates a more balanced state.[5]

For People with Eating Disorders

People with eating disorders live life out of balance. Every aspect and symptom of an eating disorder has a quality of excess: bingeing, restricting, purging, calorie counting, exercising, weighing, negative body thoughts and all the rest.

Practicing Brahmacharya, we become aware of excesses and are guided to moderate them, moving from excess into balance. In yoga postures we call this *edge*. The edge of a pose is the way of being in the posture that is not too much and not too little. In a side bend, for instance, the edge is an amount of bend that is both sustainable and challenging.

All psychotherapy should keep this concept in mind. When helping our clients we cannot push too little or too hard. We cannot force balance.

Bramacharya has to be practiced and internalized. We can impose external control of our clients' symptoms in treatment programs, for example, weight gain, or preventing purging, but unless they internalize the desire and ability to control their own thoughts and behaviors, change their focus, and find balance, the eating disorder symptoms will return. On the other hand, guiding clients to shift their focus from the over-valuation of weight and shape creates room for other more meaningful pursuits, which in turn naturally aid in the reduction of behaviors related to weight and shape goals.

Brahmacharya helps a person redirect energy away from one place and towards something else. Once there is balance, clients have more energy to focus on parts of life that need attention and healing. Psychological, emotional, and spiritual energy are available to tackle other situations, such as developing significant human relationships.

One client of mine severely out of balance, stole food and binged on food and men. She studied the concept of Brahmacharya in her eating and impulsive stealing behaviors and worked at developing a greater capacity for being in her body, feeling her feelings, and developing tolerance for intimacy. As she peeled away the layers, she realized the imbalance of her continued stealing. Over time, yoga helped her develop the skills to lean into her urge to steal without having to act on the impulse. She no longer binges on food or men or finds distraction in restriction and stealing. She continues Brahmacharya as a practice to nurture the balance in her life.

For Providers and Loved Ones

How do we balance taking care of the person with the eating disorder with taking care of our relationships and ourselves? What's enough work, and what's too much work? How many appointments should we have? How many days per week should we work? How do we balance a family or social life outside of our work?

There is no simple answer to finding balance; like life itself, balance is not a destiny but a journey, which is why yoga is a practice, not an immovable point.

Balance in life and in yoga is achieved by moving in and out of balance, by hovering in it and then losing it. A key to being in balance is paying attention and knowing when you've lost it!

Aparigraha: Non-grasping/Non-attachment

In the practice of aparigraha, we consider who we are without outer layers of accomplishments and ego. If I am not an "A" student, am I good enough? If I don't make a three-figure salary, am I worthy?

Our culture teaches that the more we accomplish, the more valid we are. We need the "A" on our paper to demonstrate that learning has occurred. On a treadmill, we feel accomplished if we have achieved our "distance" goal.

Part of Aparigraha is learning to deal with our competitiveness and desire to have what someone else has or be what someone else is. It is about learning to be happy with what we have and not coveting. It is also about not being attached to our possessions or to life going a certain way. Practicing Aparigraha, means learning how to not be attached to the results.

With Aparigraha we learn to let go. We have all had the experience of holding on too tightly to someone or something because we fear losing the things we value. However, it is our attachment that actually causes our suffering.

For People with Eating Disorders

Aparigraha provides a framework for an essential question: "Who am I without my eating disorder?" With Aparigraha, we learn to shed the layer of the eating disorder identity and imagine life without it.

An eating disorder produces a lot of comparisons, clinging and attachment. An eating disorder of any type can turn into an identity that the person becomes attached to. People easily mistake the eating disorder identity for who they really are and are afraid to give it up because they don't know who they will be without it. Recovery requires letting go of attachment to a number, food, a body size, comparisons and the eating disorder identity.

The practice of Aparigraha recently helped one of my clients (and me) take an important step forward. This client slowly made progress in increasing her calories, gaining needed weight, and releasing her grip on her eating disorder identity and her attachment to the number on the scale. And then, in one memorable session, she asked me to do the same—by weighing her less frequently. I realized that to practice Aparigraha I too would have to be less attached to the scale and agreed to weigh her monthly instead of weekly. This reminded us both not to stay attached to things that no longer serve us.

For Providers and Loved Ones

For the clinician or family member, practicing Aparigraha means the Three As:

- No Assumptions.
- No Agenda.
- No Attaching to outcome.

This might at first seem counter-intuitive, but freedom from grasping is as important for the person caring for an individual recovering from the eating disorder as it is for the person recovering. It is important to understand and validate our role in supporting someone's recovery, while staying neutral and unattached to the outcome.

For example, both family members and clinicians can hold assumptions about the identified client, cling to agendas for treatment, and attach to a particular outcome, even when all these things might not be right for the person or the right time.

There are times when an active and directive approach is necessary; for example, when the person is younger or someone is critically ill or in danger. However, a certain amount of loving detachment is needed for us not to get in the way, push an agenda, and cause too much resistance. When we are too attached to an agenda or outcome the person we are trying to help might withdraw, resist and not tell the truth.

Practicing Aparigraha, means creating an environment conducive to honesty and truth and ultimately allowing the other person to become the teacher, the one in the driver's seat, on his or her journey towards true self and a new life.

Niyamas

Niyamas are five yoga observances that foster the ethical and spiritual aspects of the self: Saucha, Santosha, Tapas, Svadhyaya and Ishvarapranidhara.

Saucha: Purity

Saucha loosely translates as "purity" or "cleanliness" and is an invitation to cleanse our bodies, attitudes and actions. Inner cleanliness is about maintaining a healthy body and mind. Outer cleanliness is about creating a healthy environment and moving towards positive behaviors and nourishing relationships.

The notion of cleansing the body can mean many things—and some interpretations can be hazardous. Saucha is sometimes associated with fasting or using juice cleanses to promote purity of the body, a set of behaviors readily misused and abused by many people, including some with eating disorders.

For People with Eating Disorders

Eating disorders are toxic to the body and spirit. In attempts to alter their weight, patients abuse coffee, artificial sweeteners, diuretics, laxatives and other substances to the point of causing harm to the workings of the body. All kinds of symptoms are seen in patients with eating disorders, including gastroesophageal reflux disease (GERD), irritable bowel syndrome (IBS), and erratic blood sugar levels.

Saucha teaches clients that inner cleanliness means not filling oneself with harmful and nutrient lacking substances, but rather, eating enough nutritious food daily, maintaining a healthy weight, and learning to replace disordered thoughts, negative self-talk, and distorted perceptions with healthy ones. Outer cleanliness means practicing self-care and creating a healthy environment conducive to becoming symptom-free and ultimately recovered.

For Providers and Loved Ones

Saucha is relevant for everyone because of the toxicity of our culture in regards to the body, self, and relationships. The principle of Saucha helps us resist dieting propaganda and the seduction of indulging in quick fixes. Practicing Saucha we can improve our environment and make it more conducive to our values. Several years ago I made a commitment to practice Saucha by disengaging from all media that encourages body dissatisfaction in men and women. I stopped watching reality television that exploits individuals with weight and eating problems and stopped reading magazines filled with airbrushed models and dieting tips. I removed from my office any magazines that could be triggering to my clients and their loved ones and replaced them with Buddhist and yoga magazines instead.

Santosha: Contentment/Acceptance

Mother Teresa said, "Be happy in the moment, that's enough. Each moment is all we need, not more." This is the spirit of Santosha, which asks us to find contentment in the present moment and acceptance of one's experience.

Santosha, (acceptance) and Satya, (truth) go together. When awareness of the *truth* is present, the opportunity opens to *accept* the experience as it is. Contentment should not be confused with happiness or complacency. It is neither. Santosha is the peace of accepting what is, like the AA serenity prayer. Accepting what is then allows us to move forward with changing the things we can. Santosha is not a state but an active practice of acceptance and contentment.

For People with Eating Disorders

Most of the time, people suffering with eating disorders are far from content. They obsess about what already happened or try to control for the possibilities of what *could* happen. The present moment is often experienced as overwhelming and symptoms serve to distract, numb, or push away the discomfort. The never-ending cycle of dissatisfaction, resistance and fear prevent contentment or acceptance.

A person struggling with binge eating who is eager to lose weight is living in non-acceptance of his or her body, which usually leads to even more binging. Often these patients give up prematurely if they don't see the number on the scale changing fast enough.

Santosha, learning to be in the present and accept what is, is an important recovery tool. In recovery, Santosha means being in an experience while feeling and tolerating discomfort—without using symptoms. This is not the same thing as being happy. In fact, there is no expectation that one will be "happy," but that the person will experience acceptance rather than resistance.

A patient of mine recently spent several months at an outpatient facility working on her binge eating disorder. After she left the program, she began to spiral into symptoms once again but could not accept or deal with it. First there was denial ("It's not that bad"), then alarm ("It's worse than I thought"), and finally, hopelessness ("I'll never get better"). It took several sessions to move through these stages into the reality of where she was and then to an acceptance of that reality. Once she accepted the reality of her symptoms *without* comparing them to past or future, she was able to respond appropriately by picking back up the tools and supports she learned in treatment. This is Santosha.

For Providers and Loved Ones

Eating disorders are devious, cunning, powerful and illogical. Recovery is not a linear process. We can become disillusioned with the disorder and frustrated with the process, no matter how much we care about the person affected. This is why Santosha is so helpful.

The well-known Serenity Prayer is a good mantra for the practice of Santosha: asking for serenity to accept the things we cannot change, the courage to change the things that we can, and the wisdom to know the difference between them.

There is a massive difference between supporting someone on the journey and dragging someone towards the destination. When impatience rises up inside me, I say to myself, "This is not my journey, it's so-and-so's." That reminds me to back off when I feel overly invested in the outcome and return to working on my own acceptance of the process.

Tapas: Fiery Discipline

The literal translation of Tapas is heat or "to burn." The concept of Tapas is to seek a burning desire or fiery self-discipline which leads to transformation. It's a powerful, but often misunderstood, observance.

Many people associate self-discipline with mastering something that is difficult. However, this is not the essence of Tapas. Just because something is difficult doesn't mean it's transformational. Although some good things are challenging, not all challenging things are good.

For People with Eating Disorders

People with eating disorder confuse their behaviors with examples of fiery discipline. Our society praises people for extreme dieting, weight loss and exercise without consideration for the consequences. In reality unbending control of what someone eats or rigid commitments to exercise may look like self-discipline but are actually obsessions that obligate the person to make certain choices. It does not take fiery discipline for someone with anorexia to skip a meal or pass up cookies, and it is a mistake to think so. Teaching the concept of Tapas is very useful since we can help patients distinguish real self-discipline from an eating disorder mindset.

For a client with an eating disorder, true fiery discipline means sticking to a meal plan instead of giving in to food restriction or bingeing. It also takes work and discipline to counter negative thoughts, move towards positive ones, consistently keep appointments, and stay focused on one's recovery.

I encourage my clients to recognize the energy they expended on restricting, the intense focus of bingeing, the discipline of exercise, and the force behind other symptoms. I offer hope by assuring them that they can and will re-channel this same Tapas energy into the process of recovery, the passion for life, and the discipline to maintain appropriate eating practices.

Tapas can help someone tap into the "burning desire" to get better.

For Providers and Loved Ones

There are moments in my work when I feel frustration with the seemingly surface vanity of the eating disorder—or of our wider shared culture. If I hear another person complain of being fat or say they can't eat, I want to respond by shouting, "Just eat!" I know that loved ones sometimes feel that way, too—and yet frustration-driven commands rarely do any good.

For practitioners, the Niyama of Tapas helps us remember why we chose to do the work we do. When we practice tapas we allow the heat of passion or burning enthusiasm to carry us in our work—rather than be misdirected into our frustration with the disorder.

Tapas can help loved ones remember and experience the passion they have for the true self of the person they love. It can ignite us to engage in self-care and commit to supporting our loved one's recovery, no matter where that journey leads.

I draw on the practice of Tapas to lead me back to my passion to be an advocate for the bodies whose voices were stolen by an eating disorder. It is when I can ignite my own fire and focus on the deeper dynamics of the eating issues that I can truly serve.

Svadhyaya: Self Study

Svadhyaya is the pursuit of knowing oneself, learning what drives us and what shapes us. It asks us to look at the stories we tell ourselves about ourselves—and realize how these stories create our reality. Ultimately, this fourth Niyama invites us to release the false and limiting self-perception that our ego imposes on us, so we can know our true selves.

Svadhyaya is hard to grasp for many people, because it is soul work—the kind of work that's very hard to put into words. Svadhyaya is often associated with meditation, but it really encompasses any activity that invites self-exploration.

There is a saying that we are not human beings having a spiritual experience, we are spiritual beings having a human experience. This aspect of Svadhyaya is worth remembering. We are not here just to learn who we are as individuals, but also to *remember* our deeper truth.

For People with Eating Disorders

As discussed earlier, people with an eating disorder frequently come to see the disorder as their identity. The symptoms of the eating disorder and the stories around it become the characteristic qualities of the individual. Recovery requires self-discovery and an end to one's attachment to the eating disorder self.

A big part of Svadhyaya's self-study is mourning the loss of the eating disorder identity. When a former client finally allowed her body to gain a healthy weight, she reported that, "I lost everything I worked so hard for." When I asked her who she might be now that "underweight" was no longer a primary characteristic, she said she wished she was dead rather than having to figure out that question. This intensely powerful reaction is very real for individuals giving up the eating disorder and trying to find themselves.

Self-study in recovery can come through reading books, participating in support groups, and/or engaging in individual therapy. Self-exploration can also grow through moving the body in dance and yoga, or in creating physical expression through art or music. Each of these modalities encompasses Svadhyaya because they help individuals explore and experience many aspects of who they are—connecting with things besides the eating disorder.

For Providers and Loved Ones

Svadhyaya helps us in our work and relationships. It involves being introspective and self-reflective.

When we can be self-aware and self-reflective, we comprehend the nature of how we relate to others, and how others relate to us. It helps us address essential and often difficult questions like:

- What do I know about myself?
- What is my part in the relationship between me and another person (e.g., someone with an eating disorder)?

The practice of Svadhyaya offers a path where we maintain a "beginner's mind" by studying and learning from our natural wisdom, from others, and from our circumstances.

It is difficult for clinicians to teach Svadhyaya without also practicing it. Svadhyaya helps us understand the dynamics of relational boundaries between professional and client, how to identify and handle transference and counter-transference, and other pitfalls involved in being a clinician. From a place of self-awareness, we can use our skills to ensure safe and healthy relationships.

Like most providers, I've had clients who decided that our personalities were not a good match, and so they ended the relationship. As a new, inexperienced practitioner, this situation left me unsettled, feeling rejected, and filled with self-doubt. Svadhyaya helps me look at all aspects of the situation, such as: a) the client's fear of connecting, b) elements of my skill set that need expansion or improvement, or c) incompatibility: the reality that my personality and style can't be a match for every client or potential client.

Practicing Svadhyaya I accept myself, my strengths and my weaknesses as they are. When challenging client interactions arise, I can see them as a learning experience for me and for the other individual.

Svadhyaya helps a loved one recognize the truth that the eating disorder "is not about you, but nevertheless does affect you." Self-awareness helps us see the ways in which symptom behavior can hijack family dynamics and "trigger" us to respond in ways that escalate the situation.

Weaving Satya's truth-seeking with Svadhyaya's self-study, loved ones can sincerely survey how the eating disorder distresses and disrupts their own lives—and how attached they might be to identifying as victims of their loved one's sickness. Self-study along with truth means becoming aware of and working on "How I am reacting to another person's eating disorder."

Loved ones need to explore the degree to which the disorder takes over their own daily routine or life. They must examine what they know about themselves in relation to the disorder, and in relation to the rest of their lives.

Svadhyaya means asking difficult questions, such as "What is my part in how the eating disorder affects me?" Do I:

- Attempt to manipulate or threaten the person into "getting well"?
- Try to control their food intake?

- Secretly snoop around for signs of symptom use or "ED tools" like laxatives?
- Pull back from family and friends to avoid eating-related conflict or embarrassment?
- Tell untruths to cover up the other person's behavior?

The behaviors listed are common, painful to acknowledge, and completely understandable reactions to a complex and devious disorder. However, neither Svadhyaya nor other yoga practices use self-study or self-assessment to assign blame or feed feelings of failure.

Genuine Svadhyaya practice leads us to clarity about our relationship with eating disorders and our loved ones who have them. It helps us see authentic truths about our own behaviors. This is important because the more clearly we see our reality, the freer we are to *respond*, rather than *react*, to the disorder itself and to the distress it causes within us. Neutral, compassionate self-assessment gives us a better understanding of our need for self-care.[6]

The Nimaya observances help us develop loving acceptance of our loved one and detachment from their disorder. In the process, we learn that one of the best uses of our energy is to engage in self-care.[7]

The practice of loving self-study integrates every other Yama and Niyama along a Svadhyaya path that moves away obstacles, liberates us, and enlarges our capacity to be of service.

Ishvarapranidhana: Celebration of the Spiritual

Ishvarapranidhana means to let go and lay all our actions at the feet of the Divine (or a source greater than ourselves). The celebration of the spiritual can be tricky since the Yamas and Niyamas are not a specifically theistic philosophy. Some yoga traditions interpret Ishvarapranidhana as devotion to a particular deity, while others take it to refer to a more abstract concept of the divine, which each person understands in his/her own way.

The essence of Ishvarapranidhana is surrender—but not passive capitulation. Ishvarapranidhana is active surrender practiced and demonstrated through devotion, trust and vigorous engagement.

For People with Eating Disorders

People who have recovered from an eating disorder often recall moments of being taken into the process of healing. It can be a moment in recovery where all the work generates a sincere trust in the process. It may be a moment when one notices that there is something bigger in play—something sacred to be reckoned with.

I've been privileged to witness moments when an individual moves into healing—and to recognize how little it has to do with what we professionals have done as therapist, nutritionist, yoga teacher, psychiatrist, or physician. That moment of opening up to healing has some element of being spiritual.

Individuals who've recovered from an eating disorder will nod yes to my description, because there is unadulterated truth to this moment that is not ours to own. Many clinicians and family members will resonate, too.

That's not to say we "outsiders" make no contribution. We can all help, guide, nudge and become part of an individual's journey. But as my favorite yoga teacher said: "When this moment of healing and transformation occurs, a third party is palpable." This third party is spirit.

Letting go and falling into the unknown of recovery and healing can generate all sorts of responses, from acknowledging that the disorder was an improbable and important teacher, to a vibrant protective approach for one's newly healthy body, to a powerful commitment to serving others.

No matter what it looks like, recovery and healing means surrendering to something bigger than ourselves.

For Providers and Loved Ones

Every single time I witness surrender, an opening to healing, I am led to my own connection to the spiritual. It's impossible to stand by and observe such things impassively. The power and profundity of being present to the process of transformation moves us into gratitude and awe for the spirit.

Even from the other side of the metaphorical couch, we clinicians, family members and friends need healing. Through the practice of Ishvara-pranidhana, we too can open up and surrender to something bigger that pulses through and around us.

In yoga we have a simple ritual at the end of a practice or class. Each person bows their head to their heart and allows a moment of gratitude for the truest of all teachers … you. What follows is the word: Namaste.

Namaste translates into: "I bow to the true teacher in myself and I bow to the true teacher in you. When we acknowledge the divine in ourselves and each other we recognize we are one."

Coda

Whoever decided to read this chapter, I ask that you read the following poem. Consider a time in your life when you did this:

> Without a thought or a word, she let go.
> She let go of fear.
> She let go of judgments.
> She let go of the confluence of opinions swarming around her head.
> She let go of the committee of indecision within her.
> She let go of all the "right" reasons.
> Wholly and completely, without hesitation or worry, she just let go.

She didn't ask anyone for advice.

She didn't read a book on how to let go.

She just let go.

She let go of all the memories that held her back.

She let go of all of the anxiety that kept her from moving forward.

She let go of the planning and all of the calculations about how to do it just right.

She didn't promise to let go.

She didn't journal about it.

She didn't write the projected date in her Day-Timer.

She made no public announcement.

She didn't check the weather report or read her daily horoscope.

She just let go.

She didn't analyze whether she should let go.

She didn't call her friends to discuss the matter.

She didn't utter one word.

She just let go.

No one was around when it happened. There was no applause or congratulations.

No one thanked her or praised her. No one noticed a thing.

Like a leaf falling from a tree, she just let go.

There was no effort. There was no struggle.

It wasn't good. It wasn't bad.

It was what it was, and it is just that.

In the space of letting go, she let it all be.

A small smile came over her face. A light breeze blew through her.

And the sun and the moon shone forevermore.

Here's to giving ourselves the gift of letting go...

There's only one guru ~ you.

Now close your eyes and call to mind a time where this happened for you. This is the practice of Ishvarapranidhana.

Namaste.

Notes

1 Lee, M. (1999) "Phoenix rising yoga therapy" in Wiener, D. (ed.) *Beyond Talk Therapy: Using Movement and Expressive Techniques in Clinical Practice* (Washington, DC: American Psychological Association), pp. 205–221.

2 Patanjali, *The Yoga Sutras of Patanjali: Translation, Transliteration, and Commentary* by Sri Swami Satchidananda (Buckingham, VA: Integral Yoga Publications, 2012).

3 Cirone, M.W. (2005). "Yoga philosophy in yoga therapy: Teaching the yamas and niyamas to women with cancer." *Yoga Therapy in Practice* 1(1): 5–6.

4 Sahi, J. (2008). "Yoga and the wounded heart." *Religion & the Arts* 12(1–3), 42–76.

5 Taneja, D. (2014). "Yoga and health." *Indian Journal of Community Medicine* 39(2), 68–72.
6 Ramaprasad, D. (2013). "Emotions: An Indian perspective." *Indian Journal of Psychiatry* 55, 153–156.
7 Sahi, J. (2008). "Yoga and the wounded heart." *Religion & the Arts* 12(1–3), 42–76.

3 The Koshas: A Guide for Accessing Authentic Self

Elyse Parcher

"Who are you?"
"What do you like/dislike?"
"What do you want?"
"How do you describe yourself?"
"What makes you YOU?"

When I ask these questions in my eating disorder groups I often get blank stares. For clients with eating disorders, identity-focused questions are quite challenging and can evoke a great deal of resistance.

These individuals have lost their sense of self. An eating disorder identity is able to provide temporary relief from the anxiety of not having a sense of self, but it also leads to a shallow life and endless despair. One goal of eating disorder recovery is to find the Self, and connect back to the soul.

How does one go about finding one's Self? This question cannot be answered with empirical evidence. The Self is a purely subjective experience, and virtually impossible to define or investigate scientifically. Nevertheless, it is human nature to strive for some kind of connection to our internal truth, because somehow we know that this connection will bring us satisfaction and fulfillment. For the eating disorder population, finding the Self can heal the breaks in one's identity that eating disorder symptoms attempt to replace.

As a person who recovered from anorexia, a clinical therapist, yoga instructor/therapist and practitioner of yoga, I have been exploring the quest toward Self-identification from numerous perspectives.

Throughout my recovery, I was drawn to yoga. It made me feel alive both on and off the mat, and was the driving force that facilitated my recovery. I am forever grateful for this gift and determined to understand its power. As a yoga instructor and yoga therapist I have learned (and continue to learn) about the philosophical principles of yoga, which guide practitioners toward understanding the universal Self, the Divine and the union between the mind, body and spirit. Yoga philosophy provides the foundation for yoga's place in eating disorder (and other) recovery, especially in terms of finding one's true self. Among yoga's ancient philosophical principles, I believe the Koshas are key.

Koshas and Self

The Koshas are a guide map to the true Self. The true Self, or pure consciousness, is a permanent, Divine, reality, where suffering ceases to exist. Suffering is the result of attachment to other layers of our being that are temporary.

The Divine Self is our unchanging, eternal, core. This core is connected with a universal force, bringing us together as One. The realization of oneness, of our connection with the Divine, is the goal of yoga.[1] Achieving this is easier said than done. The Soul or Divine Self is hidden deep beneath five other subtle layers of consciousness. In yoga these layers are referred to as Koshas. Understanding the Koshas explains what yoga feels like from the inside. The Koshas are a guide for transcending these layers to the true Self, in other words, how we connect body and mind to spirit. Like a map the Koshas help you set your goal, as well as orient you, help when you get stuck, or re-direct if you lose your way, on the path to the Divine Self, (Anandamaya) bliss, the final destination.

The Sanskrit translation for Koshas, "sheaths," suggests the idea that each layer of consciousness is influenced by an interconnected counterpart. Listed from the densest to the subtlest layers of consciousness, the five Koshas are:

1   Annamaya (physical)
2   Pranamaya (breath/energy)
3   Manomaya (mind)
4   Vijnanamaya (wisdom)
5   Anandamaya (bliss)[2]

Together, the Koshas function to give us our uniqueness and create a foundation for the development of our personalities, which, while beautiful, are not permanent. Suffering occurs as we identify with our *perceived* personality rather than the real and unchanging Self. To access the Self you must understand, work through and transcend the Koshas.

Changes or vibrations in one Kosha create a vibration in all of the Koshas, influencing every aspect of our being. For example, when the physical body is tense or stressed, the breath becomes short and shallow, and the mind is easily agitated. This disruption then ripples into the wisdom body and prevents freedom from attachment to unhealthy thoughts and behaviors, ultimately blocking the path to experiencing joy.

The Koshas are like the layers of an onion, peeled back to reveal the onion's core, just as the Koshas are transcended to find the Self. Yoga teacher and author Judith Lasater writes that transcending our layers to the Self is much like the art of sculpting. To create a beautiful piece of art, the sculptor chisels away at a block of marble, removing everything which conceals the sculpture.[3]

Yoga can be practiced anywhere at any time, making it a convenient way to connect to our pure conscious Self and relieve our suffering. For most of us, this journey takes a lifetime, but even the smallest glimpses of this experience bring us closer to true meaning and fulfillment. So while yoga is certainly not an easy journey, we continue to come back to the mat because the life it brings is incredibly worthwhile.

Yoga philosophy follows an eightfold path, also called the Eight Limbs of yoga.[4] The first two limbs, Yamas and Niyamas, outline ethical precepts and observations that guide us toward making decisions in life that promote peace with ourselves, our families and our community.[5] The remaining Limbs correspond with the Kosha layers providing a path for balancing and transcending them.[6]

1 Asana (physical postures) corresponds with Annamaya.
2 Pranayama (breath) corresponds with Pranamaya (energy).
3 Pratyahara (control of the senses) and Dharana (concentration) correspond with Manomaya (mind).
4 Dhyana (meditation) corresponds with Vijnanamaya (wisdom).
5 Samadhi (Oneness with ultimate Reality) corresponds with Anandamaya (bliss).

Applying the Koshas to Recovery from Eating Disorders

Annamaya (Physical) Kosha

The first layer of our being, Annamaya, is gross matter; the physical body comprised of the food that we eat. In translation, anna means "food," and maya means "illusion." The name refers to the typical illusion that the physical body is the Self. Individuals with eating disorders often attribute their self-worth to their appearance and/or their ability to control their body. They are caught up in the "illusion" that only through the physical body are they worthy of love and happiness. The truth is, however, that the body is going to change, and will resist any attempt to stop changing. People with eating disorders endure so much suffering because they become strongly attached to their bodies. In doing so, they dedicate their lives to fighting a hopeless battle against inevitable change.

Any eating disorder treatment center makes weight stabilization a high priority. Similarly, bringing balance to the physical Kosha is crucial for initiating the route to recovery from an eating disorder, and the journey to the Self. The physical body is the only Kosha that we can see, touch, and feel. When individuals with eating disorders inflict damage on their bodies via food restriction, binge eating, purging, etc., they essentially immobilize the vehicle that allows them to navigate through the more subtle Koshas. The interconnected relationship of the Koshas means that failing to take care of the physical body will lead to blockages in its subtler counterparts, and therefore sabotage any chance of gaining access to the Self.

Annamaya Kosha for Clients with Eating Disorders

- *Eat a balanced diet of carbohydrates, fats, and protein to promote optimal functioning of organs and body systems.* Do not use a fad diet to guide your intake of food. Work with a professional until you have mastered "conscious eating," which occurs in the Manamaya (mental) Kosha.
- *Engage in moderate exercise at an intensity level that is in balance with food consumption, and safe for any physical limitations.* Appropriate exercise keeps us healthy by strengthening our defenses against numerous ailments and diseases.
- *Practice relaxation techniques.* Relieving unnecessary tension in the body nourishes the physical Kosha, and prepares the way to channel our energy toward the goal of transcending the more subtle Koshas.
- *Meditate on the physical body.* Bring awareness to your physical sensations, body position, etc. Use this exploration to go further inward, accessing other Koshas through meditation.

Pranamaya (Energy/Breath) Kosha

Prana is the Sanskrit word for "energy," or "life force." Our first breath marks the beginning of life outside the womb, and every breath we take thereafter gives us the vital energy we need to sustain this life. Prana is therefore cultivated through the breath, and so nourishing the Pranamaya Kosha involves dismantling maladaptive breathing and re-establishing a healthy breathing practice.

A common breathing pattern among those with eating disorders is constricted breathing, or chest breathing, often associated with abdominal tension and/or poor posture. Abdominal tension may be due to anxiety or a habit of holding in the mid-section to look thinner. Individuals with eating disorders tend to have poor postures that reflect their inner experience and lack of self-esteem.[7] Abnormal breathing patterns block the energetic flow of life, and affect every layer of consciousness.

The physical body is impacted by the breath, as is the breath by the body. The breath brings oxygen to the body to support its functions, and promotes relaxation by activating the parasympathetic system of the central nervous system. Similarly, tension or relaxation in the body influences the quality and texture of the breath. Understanding this bidirectional relationship allows us to navigate through the body and breath Koshas simultaneously (e.g., relaxing the body to promote deep breathing, and/or deep breathing to relax the body) as we journey inward toward the Self.

Pranamaya Kosha for Clients with Eating Disorders

- *Breathe.* The most basic form of Yoga breathing practice is the three-part breath, or diaphragmatic breathing. The three-part breath builds energy in the body to promote optimal functioning by maximizing oxygen consumption, absorption, and efficiency. The technique involves sequencing the breath from the diaphragm to the intercostal muscles and into the lungs on the inhalation, and then reversing that direction on the exhalation. Anatomically, this pulls the diaphragm downward to expand the ribs and create more room for the lungs to take in air. Although this may seem like a simple technique, it can be difficult to master if you have maladaptive breathing patterns. Once diaphragmatic breathing becomes second nature, you may be interested in advancing to other breathing practices such as alternate nostril breathing for energetic balance, breath retention for energetic awakening, or elongated breath for relaxation. Choosing a breathing practice depends on your individual needs. For example, you may find diaphragmatic breathing to be most beneficial before and/or after meals to calm the body, facilitate digestion, and promote conscious eating. You might also find it helpful to elongate the breath with a slow-count inhale, and a slow-count exhale, to relax any physical tension in the body or chaos in the mind.

Manamaya (Mental) Kosha

Manamaya is derived from the Sanskrit word for mind. The Manamaya (mental) Kosha is the level of consciousness responsible for cognitive and emotional processing of information we receive from our five senses expressed through thoughts and feelings. This Kosha allows us to make sense of the world intellectually, but can become dysfunctional or damaged if exposed to too much, too little, and/or harmful stimulation.[8] Monitoring the information we receive through our senses largely determines the well-being of our mental body, which in turn influences our other Kosha bodies.

For example, a client with anorexia may think: "If I eat, I will get fat, and if I get fat, I won't be likable." These thoughts cause a significant amount of anxiety, which leads to constriction of the breath and tension in the body. In working through the Manamaya Kosha, yoga is similar to cognitive behavioral therapy (CBT), which understands human behavior in terms of how our thoughts, feelings and physiological reactions interact. In CBT and with Manamaya Kosha, the person identifies distorted thoughts which cause or contribute to undesirable emotions and behavior, and learns to replace them with a more rational perspective. Yoga helps us nourish the mental body by training the mind to direct its focus on positive, energizing stimuli, while filtering out that which is unnecessary, harmful, or excessive.

Manamaya Kosha for Clients with Eating Disorders

- *Feed the senses with positive stimuli.* Choose to expose all five senses to images, people, places, things and activities that make you feel good! For instance, create a list of all the positive stimuli you can think of and categorize them under the senses they nourish most. This increases awareness of these stimuli in your daily life, and widens the door for you to experience them.
- *Filter out sensory information that you don't want or need.* On the yoga mat, pick a pose that you can hold for some time (e.g., corpse pose, forward fold, etc.). Set an intention to focus your mind on one point, a "drishti" (e.g., your breath, a part of your body, a gaze, a sound, etc.). See if you can keep your mind here, acknowledging your other thoughts, but resisting any attachment to them. Off the mat, you also focus your mind to move beyond the negative, "triggering" messages received from the media and elsewhere
- *Create a mantra to guide your focus back on the path to recovery.*

Guidelines for creating a recovery mantra:

1   Describe what you would like to change about your life, and/or how you live it (e.g., "I want to be more confident" and "I want to be accepted").
2   Now simply replace the "I want..." with "I am" (e.g., "I am confident" and "I am accepted"). Use these statements as your mantra(s).
3   Journal or meditate on your mantra. Notice the emotions and images associated with it.
4   Repeat your mantra whenever you begin to doubt its truth.
5   Continuing this practice, you begin to find yourself living out those images and emotions associated with your mantra, ultimately living the life you want.

Vijnanamaya (Wisdom/Intellect) Kosha

This Kosha takes its name from the Sanskrit root word, "vijana," which means "knowing." It includes all functions of the higher mind, including judgment, discernment, consciousness, and will.

Accessing this layer of consciousness comes with the realization that our thoughts, emotions, and experiences are impermanent, and do not define who we are. Those with eating disorders often lack this wisdom, and fail to see that they are connected to a larger whole. Rather, they attach their identity to impermanent aspects of themselves such as weight or body image.

Nourishing the Vijnanamaya Kosha in eating disorder recovery involves overcoming the confusion between the material and the spiritual, and then choosing to connect to the infinite, higher Self, rather than that which is temporary and leads to suffering.[9] Strengthening this higher process of the mind that connects one to the higher Self allows people to be a witness of their experience, as opposed to remaining attached to it. The wisdom gained from healing the Vijnanamaya Kosha ultimately leads to deeper insight, and the ability to experience the world in a calm, objective manner. This helps people recovering from eating disorders begin to understand and accept themselves as unique manifestations of a higher, universal Self. They realize that they are so much more than their body or anything else that their eating disorder has led them to believe.

Vijnanamaya Kosha for Clients with Eating Disorders

- *Meditate.* Take some time at the beginning and/or end of each day to meditate and clear the mind. Meditation helps strengthen your ability to witness your experiences and make rational decisions without emotional attachment.
- *Contemplate your inner experience in relation to objective reality.* Explore your thoughts, beliefs, emotions, etc. through journaling, art, or other forms of expression, and describe how they determine your inner experience in response to a specific situation. Then consider, what factors would cause someone else to experience this same situation differently? Contemplation strengthens one's ability to become a witness, and realize that reality is neutral; it is our interpretation of reality that determines how we experience it.
- *Observe your experience in a yoga pose.* Where does your mind go? What thoughts come up for you? Where do you feel any physical sensations? Do you notice any emotions? Approach this inquiry objectively by simply acknowledging the information, and letting go of any judgment or attachment to it. Accept where you are in this pose, and let it be.
- *Join a support group.* Connecting with others in recovery has numerous benefits, one of which is realizing that you are not alone, and that others share what you are going through. This connection brings us closer to the universal, higher Self within every one of us.

Anandamaya (Bliss) Kosha

This most subtle body of the Koshas is the one surrounding the Atman (True Self). When we reach this "bliss" state of consciousness, we are fully able to understand and experience our connection to all beings. Bliss is not a passing feeling; it is independent of any stimulus or reason. Indeed, it is an unchanging state of being that has always existed, but has been buried by the other Koshas. For this reason, the Anandamaya Kosha may be the most difficult to access, especially in a world where happiness is often associated with materialistic aspects of life.[10] Bliss can only be achieved when one is present in their connection to the universal Divine. Therefore, every opportunity to access the Anandamaya Kosha relies on living in the here-and-now.

From this place, we can focus on the actual experience rather than the material outcome. Transcending this Kosha is a lifelong pursuit and very few of us ever learn to live our lives fully from this state of consciousness.

Those that are able to access and transcend this Kosha demonstrate peace and wisdom beyond that of the average person, and do not suffer at the hand of material loss.[11] Although this is the ultimate goal, a great place to start is by making a daily effort to seek spiritual experiences which bring happiness, peace, inspiration and joy.

Anandamaya Kosha for Clients with Eating Disorders

- *Spiritual understanding or devotion.* Realizing that there is more to life than the material or temporary is the crux of accessing our potential to experience "bliss." Strengthening your faith in a universal Divine will bring you closer to freedom from suffering.
- *Establish and develop meaningful relationships.* Connecting with others in a meaningful way allows you to be reminded of your innate unity with other beings. This is crucial for becoming recovered from an eating disorder. Some of the ingredients that create the most meaningful relationships include selfless service, communication, active listening, empathic understanding, emotional expression, openness to feedback and the ability to stay present during interpersonal interactions. While your eating disorder may comfort you during times when you feel alone, the comfort is only temporary, and actually drives you deeper into isolation in the end. Meaningful relationships, on the other hand, endure and truly satisfy your need for connection as they bring you closer to realizing your Oneness with others in the universal Divine.
- *Connect with nature.* Spend time in nature to escape the illusion of materialistic happiness, and realize the true joy experienced when surrounded by nature's beauty and wonder. Allow nature to teach you how to slow down, be present and find peace.
- *Meditate.* Committing to a daily meditation practice facilitates your understanding of the interrelationship and well-being of all the Koshas, and ultimately brings you closer to connecting with the true Self hidden beneath these remarkable layers of our being.

To the Eating Disorder Client

Studying the Koshas and applying the exercises can be confusing. You may not have thought much about the ways you take care of your multiple layers of Being—or even considered that you have multiple layers of Being.

The following exercise from one of my Yoga Therapy teachers, Robert Butera, shows how to monitor what you do daily to nourish each Kosha. This activity allowed me to see my relationship with each of my Koshas, and increased my awareness of how my daily interactions were affecting my

Table 3.1

Physical Body	Energy Body	Mental Body	Wisdom Body	Bliss Body
I followed meal plan.	My breath seemed shallow (modify by taking 10 minutes to practice deep breathing).	At dinner, I challenged eating disorder thoughts with healthy thoughts.	I stayed present and calm in conversation during dinner.	I did not feel connected to others (I modified this by asking questions and sharing some personal experiences).

entire Being. Simply make a chart with one column for each Kosha, and then list under each column the ways in which you were able (or not able) to "feed" that particular Kosha. As you become more acclimated to this, you can then add how you might modify your behaviors or interactions to make them more favorable for your Koshas (see the examples in Table 3.1).

Throughout recovery, your emphasis on each of the Koshas is likely to change depending on your current goals. For example, in recovery from anorexia you need to spend a considerable amount of time working on weight restoration, and therefore put greater emphasis on healing the Annamaya (physical) Kosha. Focusing on one Kosha more than another at various points in recovery helps you meet your most pressing needs. Meanwhile, remember that the interconnected relationship of the Koshas allows for the healing process to permeate through all the Koshas. When you nourish one Kosha, you nourish the others. Establishing a consistent yoga practice on and off the mat eventually removes blockages from each Kosha that separate us from the Self, bringing our entire being into harmony and peace.

Summary

Yoga literally means "to unite." The magical practice of unifying our layers of consciousness brings us home to our universal connection with the true Self. When we come home, we realize that there is more to life than our impermanent appearance or possessions. When we come home, we know that we are safe and grounded because we do not attach to anything that is likely to change.

I developed an eating disorder in an effort to establish a new identity, which drove me even further away from the truth of the Self. Yoga changed my life by bringing me home from a place where I was lost and confused. The truth is that I am the infinite Self, so are you, and so is everyone else. When I connect to this true Self, I connect to the infinite, and free myself from suffering. If I attach my identity to anything else, I get hurt.

I choose to love my true Self and nourish all the layers of my Being that surround it. I choose freedom. I choose recovery.

Notes

1 Sartain, Chris, *The Sacred Science of Yoga and the Five Koshas* (Seattle: Amazon.com/CreateSpace Independent Publishing Platform, 2012).
2 Johnsen, L. (2014). "The Koshas: 5 layers of being." Posted 7/8/2014 on *Yoga International*.   http://yogainternational.com/article/view/the-koshas-5-layers-of-being (retrieved 5/25/2015).
3 Lasater, Judith Hanson. *Living your Yoga: Finding the Spiritual in Everyday Life* (Berkeley, CA: Rodmell Press, 2000).
4 Iyengar, B.K.S. *Light on the Yoga Sutras of Patanjali* (London, UK: Thorsons, 2002).
5 See Chapter 2.
6 Sartain, *op. cit.*
7 Farhi, Donna. *The Breathing Book: Good Health and Vitality through Essential Breath Work* (New York: Holt Paperbacks, 1996).
8 Butera, Robert. *Study Guide to the Classical Yoga Lifestyle* (Devon, PA: YogaLife Institute, 2003).
9 *Ibid.*
10 *Ibid.*
11 Johnsen, *op. cit.*

4 Yoga as an Adjunctive Treatment for Posttraumatic Stress Disorder: A Conversation with David Emerson

David Emerson and Joe Kelly

People with eating disorders frequently struggle with other issues, such as addiction or anxiety. Many have a history of trauma, and some suffer from Posttraumatic Stress Disorder, or PTSD. In striking recent research, trauma expert Bessel A. van der Kolk, MD and his colleagues conducted a randomized controlled trial to test yoga's impact on women with chronic, treatment-resistant PTSD. (PTSD is a type of anxiety disorder which may develop after a person is exposed to one or more traumatic events, such as child abuse, sexual assault, war, and/or serious injury.)

Sixty-four women were randomly assigned to participate in one of two groups. One group received weekly one-hour trauma-sensitive yoga classes for 10 weeks. The control group received weekly one-hour supportive women's health education for 10 weeks. At the conclusion, 52 percent of the women in the yoga group no longer met criteria for PTSD. By comparison, only 21 percent of the women in the control group no longer met PTSD criteria.

The study[1] found: "Both groups exhibited significant decreases in PTSD symptoms during the first half of treatment, but these improvements were maintained in the yoga group, while the control group relapsed after its initial improvement." They concluded that "yoga may improve the functioning of traumatized individuals by helping them to tolerate physical and sensory experiences associated with fear and helplessness and to increase emotional awareness and affect tolerance."

Experienced Registered Yoga Teacher David Emerson created the yoga model used in the study and oversaw its implementation at the Justice Resource Institute's Trauma Center in Boston. He is also a co-author of the research study, "Yoga as an Adjunctive Treatment for Posttraumatic Stress Disorder."[2] David's book, *Trauma Sensitive Yoga in Therapy: Bringing the Body into Treatment,* [3] was released in February 2015.

David spoke with co-editor Joe Kelly about the research findings, how he brings yoga to people with severe trauma, and potential insights for treating eating disorders.

Joe Kelly: How does trauma-sensitive yoga influence people with treatment-resistant PTSD?

David Emerson: We're trying to fill a void in treatment for complex trauma, or treatment-resistant PTSD. First, for the context of our conversation, let me be clear that in our program, every person who does Trauma-Sensitive Yoga (TSY) with us is also receiving psychotherapy.

In the big picture, one of the shortcomings of psychodynamic psychotherapy or psychoanalysis has been that the body is pretty much ignored. Almost all of the attention goes to the processes of thinking and talking.

In our view, and in the view of many, the body needs to be part of the treatment process. We have to actively and purposefully engage the body. Over the past 10 to 15 years, we've had modalities like sensory motor psychotherapy and somatic experiencing that have added a great deal to the process of bringing the body into treatment. Our model is in that line with sensory and somatic modalities, but there are some pretty important distinctions. The most important distinction being that with TSY, there is no attempt to *process* trauma. Basically, the mechanism we're most interested in is interoception.

JK: Can you explain interoception? I ask is because interoceptive awareness is one of the main scales on the Eating Disorder Inventory used to evaluate a client's eating disorder symptoms.

DE: Interoception, along with exteroception and proprioception, is a concept articulated about a century ago by the neurophysiologist and Nobel laureate, Charles Scott Sherrington. Interoception is our capacity to feel and sense our body's experience. It's our sense of the physiological condition or environment of the body, e.g., our perception of sensation and muscle dynamics. In the words of functional neuroanatomist A.D. Craig, interoception is our experience of our "sentient self."

Exteroception is how we perceive the stuff that's happening beyond our body in the outside world; things we can hear and see. Proprioception is why we don't walk into walls more often. It's our sense of the relative position of our body parts and how we perceive the strength of effort we use in moving those parts.

Because of advances in neuroimaging, we now know that particular parts of the brain involved in interoception are under-active in traumatized people. The next step is to figure out what methods and/or treatments might help people *reactivate* these interoceptive pathways. We think that TSY is one of them.

JK: The research paper suggests that information about one's internal milieu is a prerequisite for accurate identification of triggered emotional responses, such as fear. Why is that information so important?

DE: One idea among some of us is that identifying triggered emotional responses will help our clients tolerate discomfort, regulate their affect, and engage in less harmful behaviors.

For me, the more important things about TSY revolve around interoception and choice-making. I can understand that affect tolerance happens in TSY because people say things like, "Wow, doing TSY, I notice a level of discomfort in my body that I haven't felt before. But I also notice that I can take a few breaths or I can stop doing this form [or asana] altogether and the discomfort goes away."

This is speculation, but I believe that building the capacity to tolerate affect is more about the present moment experience of relating to your body than it is about thinking about the past and planning for the future. When someone has a flashback and then feels a rapid heartbeat and sweaty palms, their body experience is in the moment. We can learn to experience the moment and let it inform us about our immediate choices. Learning how to be aware of and present with your feelings in the moment actually helps you transform them. Living is always, in part, a present moment endeavor.

Unlike dialectical behavior therapy (DBT) or most mindfulness practices, we're not giving people skills to take home and practice. We don't do any homework or encourage any kind of *future* thinking. We're trying to help people have a true *present* moment experience with their body.

If we're right, and what is happening in TSY is mostly about interoception, then people are essentially rewiring their brain to experience the present moment (what's happening in the body right now), and then interact with it in some way (breathe or change the form) that can serve to increase affect management.

JK: How does this relate to interoception and accurate identification of the triggered emotional responses?

DE: One formulation of interoception suggests that it starts as "afferent information"—a body sensation transmitted by afferent nerves to the brain. The transmission is followed by our intrinsic attraction or aversion to the resulting emotion—known as emotional valance. Next, we have a behavior in relation to it (i.e. moving toward or away from a stimulus).

In trauma-sensitive yoga, we focus on staying with the visceral afferent information, the body feeling. It's about one's capacity to sense one's body and interact with it just as it is.

As a non-clinician, frankly, I'm not interested in emotions. In the context of treating trauma, that may sound strange. However, after years of doing TSY with people with trauma, I believe it's primarily about the body experience.

I know how and why clinicians are interested in emotions. But, that's not what we do in TSY. Of course, as I said earlier, some therapy modalities do actively and purposefully engage the body—for example, sensory motor psychotherapy and somatic experiencing. However, both tend to interpret body experiences through an emotional lens. It is ultimately about the emotional response to your body and how you manage that response.

For TSY, it's not. The only thing we do is practice feeling our body. By the way, we're also really honest with clients about the fact that we *don't* always feel things—and that feeling something is not required. Choices about what to do with one's body can be made without any interoceptive experience. The client may say: "I'm just going to lift my arms to my shoulders instead of over my head, even though I don't know exactly why." That's still a valid choice and a good place to start.

Ultimately, however, we're hoping for people to connect their body experiences (interoception) with choices they're making about what they do with their body. The "I feel this, therefore, I'm going to do this" pattern becomes the feedback loop between body sensation and choices.

The feedback loop breaks down in trauma—where the pattern may be something like, "I can't feel anything, so I just do all these dangerous things."

For example, almost every youth I've worked with has scars on their arms, from cutting or burning themselves regularly and ritualistically. Somewhere along the line, there's a disconnection between their internal landscape and their behavior, between what they can feel and what they do. In that state, they're just exploring around, trying to figure out what to feel and what to do.

And, if that's the case, if we're just groping around trying to feel something and trying to manage this body that is so foreign and unknowable, then we're going to get into some seriously dangerous situations—understandably. I'm curious about whether the same thing happens in the eating disorder world.

JK: Well, eating disorder behaviors can certainly be seen as a form of self-harm. Are you saying that it's enough to have a working feedback loop—learning the body experience and then making an intentional choice?

DE: It's enough, but, again, I don't think it stands alone for everyone. In our study, we looked at people who, for three years or more, had been in talk therapy for PTSD. Nevertheless, they still qualified for the diagnosis of PTSD. This persistent diagnosis despite years of therapy is known as "treatment-resistant PTSD," which can also be characterized as complex trauma. We added 10-weeks of TSY, where these individuals worked to reconnect elements of the interoception feedback loop.

At the end of the study, more than half of the TSY group didn't have PTSD symptoms anymore at a given assessment point. What we can say is that adding trauma-sensitive yoga to "treatment as usual" had this measurable impact.

That doesn't mean they're cured; PTSD doesn't work that way. Also, I bet you that some people did start talking more about trauma with their therapists, while others didn't. I hope that someday an intern or grad student can interview the therapists and ask about how the client's relationship to therapy changed or not while they were doing TSY.

JK: When discussing TSY, you've emphasized the importance of the relationships in the healing process. Can you talk about that?

DE: Relationships involve, among other things, power dynamics. As *Trauma and Recovery* author Judith Herman says, trauma itself is largely about power dynamics within relationships.[4] Her suggestion, and one that we take very seriously with TSY, is that trauma *treatment* is also about working out power dynamics within relationships. Herman calls this *empowerment*.

For us, empowerment is about who is in control of this body. We focus on turning over control to the people we're working with. We do this by giving our students choices, real choices, about what they want to do with their body in a given yoga form.

Yoga forms are wonderful opportunities to experiment with empowerment because they offer so many options, so many opportunities to make choices about what to do. You can put your arm like this, or like that, or over there. Somebody who is new to yoga, and really symptomatic, can do just a couple of choices. When people get a bit more interested in their body and have more curiosity and interoceptive ability, then we can offer more complex options for them to choose from.

This is in contrast to most yoga classes, by the way, which are not very choice-based. They tend to be command oriented. That's a pitfall that *we* have to be cautious about—it's tempting to just tell people what to do, for expediency or our own need to control outcomes. But that command orientation totally undermines the practice of empowerment.

So, in trauma-sensitive yoga, it's imperative to give the power of choice to the people we work with. We've learned this over the years as we've refined TSY. In the past, clients wouldn't come if we didn't give them consistent choices. Or else, they'd come and then dissociate and double down on their trauma symptoms.

It was quite painful to notice that by telling people what to do with their body—even in the slightest way—we were inadvertently reinforcing the trauma paradigm. Luckily, our clients gave us feedback on their experience, which helped us to learn our choice-based approach and to stick with it.

JJK: The reaction you describe makes sense, and I can also understand a teacher's desire to, in effect, say: "Do this because I know it will help."

DE: I'm sure it's the same with eating disorders—probably the worst thing you can do is to tell people: "Just stop doing this to your body. You're hurting yourself, so don't do it anymore." It's obviously insane for anyone trying to treat these complex issues to say things like that! But nonetheless, it's tempting, because, whether we're a friend or a treatment professional, we want to help.

It turns out though that telling a person with complicated PTSD what to do is itself traumatic. The way it is experienced by clients is: "You are controlling my body and, just as I suspected, I have no control over this thing; this body is a foreign entity. It doesn't belong to me. Why bother."

Our model is about turning over control in a purposeful and a safe way. We work together with the person to find what is the right amount of choice for him or her, what is tolerable. This client-teacher collaboration is another important aspect of relationships.

JK: Does the yoga experience need to be integrated with other parts of treatment like individual therapy?

DE: As I mentioned earlier, everyone who does TSY with us is also in traditional, talk therapy. We have found that many people, not all but many, need to be able to talk about their TSY experiences with a skilled professional who understands trauma. So we do work as part of a team.

JK: Do you mean to say that some people don't necessarily need to process TSY with their therapist?

DE: What typically happens is that people come into the yoga session, and when we do some form, there's a trauma trigger. The person's implicit memory is triggered.

At that point, as a TSY facilitator, my job is to keep the experience oriented to the body in the present moment. In other words, we stick with the physical experience in the form, "notice what you feel in these muscles," and we work with that through choice. We say things like: "would you like to try and change the form a little bit and how does that feel now?" or "would you like to come out of this form entirely and try something else?"

We want to give people the chance to interact with their actual body experience as it is, and to possibly make some changes to what they are experiencing in their body, based on what they do with their body. That's the empowerment issue we discussed earlier. Later, if they find it necessary, they can talk with their therapist about any trauma-related content that may have surfaced during the yoga forms. Talking about that while doing the forms would take away from our goal: getting the person out of his or her mind and into his or her body.

That's really where we're coming from in terms of our understanding of trauma. It's a body thing. It's a present moment body thing. And, so we teach our clients how to meet the distressing experience or any body experience not by *thinking* about trauma but by *interacting* with what is happening in their body. For some people that's enough and that's fascinating to me.

JK: So, why is "that's enough" so fascinating to you?

DE: First of all, because I studied to become a clinical social worker for a little bit, but never really quite "got" talking. During my own experience in therapy, I never really felt like I was getting much from talking. The talk wasn't comfortable for me. I see people who are good at it, and I don't mean to say that talk therapy isn't effective; it just wasn't comfortable for me.

And so the idea that you can do clinically relevant work without talking, without processing, is pretty interesting.

I want to be really clear and say that this approach is not for everybody. There are people who have to process their experiences, and there are also people who don't. We ought to be cautious about requiring verbalization.

Clinically relevant non-verbal work is a pretty encouraging possibility, especially when we come to complex trauma. Because we know that, in traumatized people, the parts of the brain which let us verbally articulate our experience are compromised or under-active.[5]

Take for example young soldiers and Marines who come back from war. Many are still adolescents—and they are traumatized. They *literally* can't talk about their trauma. If talk therapy is the only option, they're going to be stuck, self-medicating, or worse, until they can figure out words for their trauma, which may or may not ever happen. Or, they can start doing some clinically relevant treatment that doesn't require words, and does address the PTSD symptoms. I think it's very encouraging that there's a possibility for treatment that is not language based.

JK: That's one of the impressive things about the findings, especially because complex trauma seems so intractable.

DE: I agree. And we studied cases of extremely complex trauma. My sense is that people have the same fear of eating disorders that they have of complex trauma. They're afraid that, because it's so intractable, there's nothing we can do.

JK: And understandably so. Many people live with eating disorders for decades and either don't get help, or periodically get help that does or does not provide some temporary relief, and then they're back into symptom use again. It involves eating and it's a body thing, so it's about body experience, disconnection, disregulation, and power and control, too. Like getting drunk or cutting, a binge or purge can provide temporary numbing. Plus, people with eating disorders often do abuse substances, self-injure, suffer from PTSD, and have other mental illnesses. It's very complicated.

DE: For me, the key response to the complexity is learning from our students. People tell us what they need and what's happening, and it's incredible. For instance, it's common to hear people say: "The reason I'm coming in here is because I can't let my kids touch me" or "any intimacy with my partner is intolerable."

JK: Why is that scenario so common?

DE: Because that's what Complex Trauma is. Bessel van der Kolk does a very good job of articulating this. Trauma is not being able to hold the hand of your lover or snuggle on the couch. It's not even being able to hold your kids. These are things that humans want the most. We want to be able to be held and to hold. And when we are traumatized these human things become excruciating.

Reckoning with these physical experiences is so important for treating trauma. When a client says: "That's where my pain is" and the psychotherapist says: "Let's *talk* about it," it can feel like a huge disconnect to the client. People with complex trauma don't feel safe in their body. Their experience is: "What's actually happening?" and "I don't have a body that's predictable or safe." We can either talk about that or we can practice interacting with this body that doesn't feel predictable and safe. What we do with TSY addresses that dilemma in a very concrete way.

JK: It seems clear that trauma-sensitive yoga is different than yoga people encounter elsewhere. You have talked about some of those differences, but are there any others?

DE: For starters, we don't do physical assists. No hands-on touching to assist people. We learned very clearly how destructive it was. Touching by the teacher especially damaged the person's relationship to themselves, as well as our relationship with them.

In our model, people get to practice being completely in charge of their body. Many times, we heard people in the study say "I don't know quite why, but now I *can* let my kids touch me" or "My partner and I started to talk about sex in our couple's therapy, and that's really the key issue we've never talked about before."

So, the speculation is that developing a relationship with your own body—a relationship that revolves around interoception and choice—allows people to reach a point where they genuinely believe: "I feel safe enough in my body and, therefore, I can let other people touch me where and when it's appropriate."

This kind of response from our clients strengthens my personal sense that interoception and choice are the keys to the effectiveness of TSY. What do I feel? What do I not feel? What can I do? What can I not do? How do I change this? These are the things that make me feel like I can have relationships that aren't out of control.

JK: Tell us more about the no-touching approach. How did you learn what you learned about physical assists being destructive for people with complex trauma?

DE: The yoga community and teachers in the West are kind of obsessed with touching students and providing physical assists. If you go to a typical yoga class, the teacher will probably touch you or somebody near you and adjust your body in some way. Sometimes teachers ask if they can, other times they don't ask. That's a crap shoot. But the idea is that there's a lot of touching going on in yoga. The teacher, the person in power, is touching you.

When I say this in the context of trauma, which includes the trauma of physical and sexual abuse, most people cringe.

The people who don't cringe think that their students need to learn how to be touched in a safe way. They have this idea that, "If they come to yoga class, and I can touch them safely, then they'll learn to be touched safely, and their trauma will be eased."

I would suggest that the opposite is happening for people with trauma, because ultimately the most important relationship when dealing with trauma is *my* relationship to *my* self, *my* body. It's not about me feeling safe with you—the teacher and person in power—touching me. As soon as you place your hands on somebody, it creates a very clear power dynamic: I (the teacher) am in charge of your (the student's) body.

We learned, through feedback from our clients, that when the teacher touched the student, it wasn't creating safety. Instead, it was making people feel like they're doing something wrong, that they couldn't trust what they were feeling in their own body, that they don't have any choices, and that they aren't in charge of their body. A major conflict was created: clients wanted to do a certain thing with their body and the teacher was making them do something else. This took away safety in the relationship. It was disempowering.

I've had yoga teachers try to convince me that "I don't do it that way; I'm very gentle and very caring and a very intuitive person." And that may all be true, but in this context, when we're dealing with complex trauma, that's not how you're perceived.

People are afraid of you. They are distrustful of you, *especially* if they like you. They're horrified of their body and what you think of their body. All that stuff is way more powerful than how nice you think you are.

At first, we didn't know what we were doing and, like many yoga teachers, we didn't want people to feel untouchable. We came from a good place, but didn't yet understand just how touch is experienced dynamically by a person with complex trauma. We were looking at it from the outside, not the inside. For that person with trauma, how gentle or intuitive I think I am is irrelevant. It's what I do that matters.

JK: What qualities would you most value and be looking for in a yoga teacher when it comes to dealing with complex trauma?

DE: First is some knowledge about what complex trauma is. Someone who is caring enough about the subject to learn what's out there and what the research is. Learn how people understand the particular affliction you're dealing with. That knowledge will support yoga teachers quite a bit.

Then, just being open to not having a rigid idea about what yoga is. We have enough inflexibility out there, where some teachers adopt the approach of: "I learned yoga from this particular lineage, and this is how I'm going to do it and teach it. Period." In light of what you learn about complex trauma, you need the flexibility to adjust some of what you learned about yoga.

I look for a yoga teacher who is willing to listen to people, whether students or colleagues. It needs to be someone who is able to listen and respond appropriately and make changes where appropriate. In short, the same kind of qualities you want in a good therapist.

Ideally, yoga teachers wouldn't be going it alone on this. I believe TSY should be done as part of a team, where the yoga teacher has regular consultation with clinical people—and vice versa. Ideally, those lines of communication go both ways.

JK: Is this model being replicated anywhere outside of Boston?

DE: A paper was published in 2014 by researchers at the University of Minnesota who studied TSY with women in a domestic violence program. There's another group we're consulting with now at Emory University. They're working with the Atlanta VA Medical Center, doing a feasibility study with women who've experienced military sexual trauma. So far, the studies all have female cohorts, which is a limitation. I hope someone can take this work and use it with men, and see what they get. For our part we do trainings for clinicians and yoga teachers and have an annual certification program for yoga teachers in our model.

Additional Resources:

- *Overcoming Trauma through Yoga: Reclaiming Your Body* by David Emerson and Elizabeth Hopper, PhD (Berkeley, CA: North Atlantic Books, 2011).
- *The Body Keeps the Score: Brain, Mind, and Body in the Healing of Trauma* by Bessel van der Kolk, MD (New York: Viking, 2014).

Notes

1 Van der Kolk, B.A., Stone, L., West, J., Rhodes, A., Emerson, D., Suvak, M. and Spinazzola, J. (2014) "Yoga as an Adjunctive Treatment for Posttraumatic Stress Disorder: A Randomized Controlled Trial." *Journal of Clinical Psychiatry* 75(0). http://ww.traumacenter.org/products/pdf_files/Yoga_Adjunctive_Treatment_PTSD_ V0001.pdf(accessed 11/16/15).
2 Ibid.
3 Emerson, D. (2015) *Trauma Sensitive Yoga in Therapy: Bringing the Body into Treatment*. New York: W.W. Norton & Company.
4 Herman, J. (2015) *Trauma and Recovery: The Aftermath of Violence—From Domestic Abuse to Political Terror* (New York: Basic Books).
5 van der Kolk, Bessel (2014) *The Body Keeps the Score: Brain, Mind, and Body in the Healing of Trauma* (New York: Viking).

5   Yoga and Samskaras: Breaking Through Eating Disorders Patterns

Lauren Peterson

In 1996 I was making my living as a yoga teacher. Earlier in my life I had been a professional ballet dancer and had suffered from anorexia. Yoga had helped me recover. Each year I taught, I saw an increasing number of students coming to classes who were obviously suffering like I had, starving their bodies and their souls, but searching for something in yoga. When Carolyn Costin asked me to bring yoga to Monte Nido, the residential program she was opening for eating disorders, I was intrigued and knew it was a calling. I believed I had a lot to offer with my personal background and my extensive yoga training.

Neither Carolyn nor I knew of any other eating disorder centers offering yoga, so we had no precedents or guidelines to follow. Back then, and again recently when asked to write a chapter for this book on yoga and eating disorders, a few main questions came to mind:

- What is yoga?
- What is the goal of having a yoga practice?
- What exactly is a yoga practice?
- How can yoga help people with eating disorders?

Yoga means "union" and the purpose of yoga is to unite: body to mind and us to the experience of life. If you think of yoga only as a form of exercise, this definition might confuse you. Of course, some forms of yoga do take place in gyms, but the physical yoga we see in classes or videos is only a small part of the picture. Some practices of yoga don't involve physical exercise at all. They are centered on study, or work, or devotion. In my work at Monte Nido and in this chapter, I focus on "hatha" yoga, which begins as a physical practice, but doesn't end there. I wanted to help bring the deeper elements of yoga that had helped me into the work Carolyn was doing with clients. I knew the kinds of things I could teach and bring to an overall approach to recovery involving body and mind.

Hatha yoga is a system of working the body, through postures (asanas) and the breath (pranayama) to explore deep-seated patterns, habits, and conditioning of the mind. It is exactly this conditioning of the mind that yoga can target and begin to bring new awareness to. Through yoga we can develop new perspectives and change old, entrenched behavior patterns (such as those found in people with eating disorders).

Samskaras

All of us develop conditioned responses to what happens within and around us. Yoga teaching calls these responses Samskaras. In Sanskrit, "sam" means "to collect together" and "kara" refers to repeated patterns, things, activities, or deeds. "Samskaras" can be translated as deeply held patterns, conditioning, or habits collected in the body.

Once we develop insight into our Samskaras, we can see who we are separate from our Samskaras. Being able to experience ourselves, in the moment, apart from any long developed habits or conditioning is the ultimate goal of any complete yoga practice.

We come into the world completely dependent beings, needing to be held, clothed and nurtured. We feel hunger, are fed, and stop eating when we are full. As newborns, we are pure observers, without prejudice or judgment. Like sponges, we soak up information. We have no perception of ourselves as attractive or not. In fact, we have no body image at all. We have only body experience—laughter, crying, hunger, peeing, feeling full, sleeping, cuddling, etc. We have no "preconceived" ideas about who or what we should be.

As we grow, we pick up ideas about right and wrong, good and bad, and what is attractive and desirable. Cultural and societal norms play a role. Our parents, schoolmates, siblings, teachers and media all influence us.

External influences affect our behavior, choices, and perspective every day. For instance, look through your old photos or scrapbooks; you'll see how ever-fluctuating fashion trends influenced what you considered attractive or desirable. Even if your hairstyle or clothes were the height of fashion back then you're likely to laugh (or cringe) at how awful that "look" would be if you wore it today.

From infancy, we also start to develop feelings and form opinions about things like food, alcohol, sex, religion, music and sports. Every person has emotional responses to some (if not all) of these. Many of these responses develop at an early age.

For example, when my nephews, ages four and six, see a banner from the University of Southern California, they boo and hiss. The boys already see USC Trojans as the enemy, the team to beat. This emotional reaction is a learned response from watching their mother, who attended and worked for UCLA, the crosstown archrival of USC.

As we grow out of childhood, we can accept or reject some of our learned responses, like team allegiance. But many learned responses are more subtle and harmful than loyalty to a sports team.

Eating Disorder Behavior as Samskaras

Some people use food, drugs or alcohol as coping mechanisms to deal with pain, stress, emotional discomfort or other psychological disturbances. As these responses develop into habitual patterns or Samskaras they can grow into addictions or compulsive eating patterns. Over-eating, over-drinking, or using drugs may "work" to give an immediate and temporary fix for our distress. However, these coping strategies do not really solve the sources of our distress—and they often become problems themselves. As addictions and compulsions grow, shame, guilt and remorse usually follow.

Over-indulgence is not the only form of compulsion or learned response to stress. In today's culture where controlling one's food and figure is highly valued among females, many exert rigid, restrictive control over their food intake, finding a false sense of satisfaction and control. Adolescent girls are especially vulnerable because their bodies are changing beyond their control and they don't know what they will look like when fully mature. There are many reasons for the development of an eating disorder but known factors include restricting food in order to gain control, obtain the idealized body, and mitigate the developmental upheaval of puberty.

In our society, the ability to restrict eating is often revered. People long to be thinner, go on and off diets, and ravenously consume magazines bursting with diet tips. In this environment, a girl feels powerful, in control and more desirable when she restricts her food intake and loses weight. Sadly, this restriction pattern can become a compulsion over which she loses control.

If you have a healthy relationship with your body, you listen and respond to signals that your body sends out. How does someone learn the necessary appropriate healthy responses?

Ideally, children are given food when they cry from hunger, affection when they need comfort, and safe places to explore and be curious. Through appropriate caregiving, children learn to trust their ability to recognize their needs, and find healthy ways to fulfill them. Through stimulating play, healthy food and appropriate responses to their needs, children learn the value and purpose of their body setting them on a path towards a healthy body and a good relationship with their body.

At the other extreme, dieting to look a certain way or fit into someone's idea of beauty teaches people to ignore communication from their bodies— even hunger pains. Compulsive eaters lose touch with the body's fullness signals, designed to guide us on how much and how often to eat. Binge eaters gorge food in unhealthy amounts, not even enjoying it. People with anorexia nervosa will ignore the body's need for food, up to and beyond the brink of starvation. The common thread here is that people with eating disorders lose their ability to recognize and respond to body signals. Yoga helps many people (including me) heal from their eating disorder by reconnecting body and mind to work together again, appropriately recognizing and responding to each other's signals.

When healthy and content we eat for both pleasure and nourishment, and stop eating when full and sated. Just as we fill a car when it is running low on gas, stopping the pump before the tank overflows, we naturally sense the cues to ingest the amount of energy needed to maintain healthy body functions.

Unfortunately due to a variety of risk factors, too numerous and complicated to describe in this chapter, some people intertwine emotional issues with food, eating and body image. They essentially fiddle with their body's "fuel gauge," ignoring cues and restricting, overeating and purging. Over time, these patterns are locked deep into both brain and body consciousness and they becoming habitual patterns or Samskaras. Eventually, the "fuel gauge" stops functioning and—like a car whose dashboard gauges short out—these individuals risk danger. The first step to getting rid of Samskaras is to recognize them. A yoga practice can help.

Using Yoga to Help Heal Eating Disorders

The first step to eliminating harmful habits is to recognize them—which is a skill yoga helps people develop by continually bringing awareness to the present moment. The important thing for recovery is to teach yoga techniques to students or clients in class, while consistently helping them learn how the techniques can be applied to life off the mat. Most people go through their days fairly unconscious of the habits or patterns they're following. Some habits like waking up, fixing breakfast and taking the bus to work, help us navigate life without exerting excessive energy. Other habits, like bingeing and purging, smoking, or drinking, can hurt us.

Yoga consistently reinforces being in the present moment—standing in our bodies, taking air in, breathing air out. As we move through postures in hatha yoga, we are looking for a combination of steadiness (shira) and ease (sukha). Steadiness is important in helping us go through our lives confident, assured and strong. Ease is also important so we relax into every moment, practicing acceptance, helping us to handle challenges or setbacks. When you are at ease, in acceptance, you can take a step back, get a new perspective, and see things more clearly. This isn't easy at first, especially for people struggling with disconnection from their bodies, distortion about their selves and patterns of emotional dysregulation.

Even the healthiest, most emotionally balanced yoga beginners may have difficulty when first attempting a yoga posture (asana). For example, in the seated hip opener, or "double pigeon," your hips may tense up initially, resisting the stretch. You may not be able to extend your knees very far or do the pose comfortably. A good teacher will help you make personal adjustments suited to you and your body. This is yoga: you and your body, together finding the way. In yoga the "inability" to do a pose in a certain prescribed way is not a failure—or a reason to give up. Practicing yoga means exploring the pose and going further at your own pace.

During your first minute in double pigeon pose, there will be a lot of resistance in your muscles. You will come to a true understanding of your range of motion in the posture. You will also understand that your range of motion can improve with time and practice. To take any posture to the next level, you need to stay with it, breathing and relaxing into the pose. Once you learn this you will be able to apply this technique to other resistance in your life (emotional, psychological, spiritual and/or social).

It is possible, and even common, to go through yoga poses on autopilot. For example, once you have been doing yoga for a while, you might do a pose without paying much attention to your body and how it is feeling and moving. However, a good yoga teacher will help guide you, remind you to pay attention to your breath, your body and come to awareness inside.

Going into autopilot doesn't mean failure. With practice and guidance, we bring ourselves back and reconnect with the true practice of yoga. We dig deep into recognizing the present moment, perceive our sensations, and then respond to them with intention and patience—just like we allow the resistance to melt away in double pigeon.

Taking New Samskaras from the Mat to Daily Life

As I watched those first eating disorder clients develop a yoga practice, I found them increasingly striving to be more in the moment and present off the mat and in their recovery. We would have discussions on how they could more easily separate themselves from their old habits and identity. They became more mindful of old conditioned responses and the power they had to change them. They grew more hopeful and willing to eliminate what was not truly serving them.

We all shared how difficult it was to change habitual patterns but how yoga helps through its reminders about being in the moment and accepting ourselves, while nurturing the willingness to nudge ourselves into necessary change. I was struck by how much I saw yoga help the clients begin to listen to their bodies, help them actually be in their bodies, and even honor their physical selves. In some cases clients even said that their cravings and desire for the old behaviors decreased and in some cases even melted away. This had been the case for me—and was a key part of becoming recovered from my eating disorder. I was profoundly grateful that I was now helping others do the same. Many of the clients expressed a desire to continue yoga upon discharge and we helped them set up a yoga practice as part of their ongoing care. I still hear from clients who say that yoga was an integral part of their recovery process.

It was then, and is still today, rewarding and astonishing to see how so many eating disorder clients take to yoga and seem to benefit in the same ways that yoga helped me. I can still remember yoga's effect on my own healing journey. It kept me returning to the present and replaced destructive patterns that fed my anorexia. Getting in touch with my body taught me to pay attention in new ways. I learned what my body really craved—and what my heart and soul craved too: connection, acceptance and meaning.

I learned new responses to life, new Samskaras. I learned to eat a healthy, balanced diet while not forbidding any food. I stabilized in a weight range that supports healthy body function. My body became more muscular and strong, my period returned, and thankfully, blessedly, I eventually became pregnant and gave birth to a beautiful baby boy. In addition to eradicating my eating disorder and making me strong and physically healthy, my yoga practice continues to make me a better and more patient mother, friend and teacher.

Hatha yoga brought together the physicality that I so enjoyed when I was a dancer with the spiritual path of self-awareness that I had been seeking. Ultimately, yoga taught me to enjoy the richness of all my experiences. This doesn't mean I live a life without disappointment or hardship, but I have the tools to navigate challenges and continue on. As the first yoga teacher at Monte Nido treatment center, I repeatedly witnessed how, as it did for me, yoga taught people with eating disorders to be in their bodies, increase self-acceptance, face their issues, and approach life with more steadiness, ease and an open heart.

As the great James Baldwin wrote back in 1962: "Not everything that is faced can be changed, but nothing can be changed unless it is faced."[1]

Note

1 Baldwin, J. (1962), "As Much Truth as One Can Bear" in *The New York Times Book Review*, January 14, p. 38.

6   Yoga and Eating Disorders: What the Research Does and Doesn't Say

Tosca Braun, Tamar Siegel and Sara Lazar

Eating disorders have adverse effects on mental, behavioral, psychological and physical health that engender significant suffering for patients and their families. These pernicious effects motivate persistent efforts to develop efficacious treatments.

Many eating disorder patients report disconnection from their bodies as central to their illness. Hence, therapeutic modalities that promote increased awareness of the body and the mind-body connection may be particularly relevant to this group.

Yoga is one such modality and a growing number of inpatient and outpatient treatment settings use it as an adjunct to standard therapy. Reflecting this trend, a small but increasing body of research aims to investigate the effects of yoga on eating disorders and related conditions.[1]

Inhabiting the Body

The belief that self-worth and value depend on physical appearance is common in the US, where a toned, lithe and youthful physique is a powerful cultural ideal. This belief encourages excessive emphasis on self-objectification, i.e., perceiving one's body as an object or ornament. Viewed as an object, the body becomes different from, or other than, one's subjective sense of self.

The theory of a mind-body split in eating disorders is supported by research suggesting low rates of emotional awareness,[2,3] poor interoceptive (body) awareness[4] and high self-objectification[5] in eating disordered patients. One author suggests that "active re-embodiment" is a necessary prerequisite for eating disorder recovery, and therefore recommends body-based practices that facilitate body awareness as adjunctive treatment.[6]

Yoga aims to integrate the various aspects of mind, body and spirit that comprise the self. Yogic practices such as mindfulness, self-compassion, breathing, deep relaxation and movement provide the practitioner with experiences of embodied subjectivity. Yogic philosophy contends that the body has its own wisdom, emotions, experiences and needs; yogic practices strive to cultivate awareness that the body is an important dimension of the self.[7] Learning to inhabit the body with awareness and kindness is a radically unusual experience for people with eating disorders, but one that may very well be critical for recovery.

Because research in this area is fairly new, it is important to note that little of the research has been conducted with eating disorder patients. In addition, the existing research does not use methods or designs that allow us to say with certainty that yoga directly influences eating disorders and its symptoms. The following sections discuss research on yoga for eating disorders/behaviors as well as research related to areas of special interest and/or high relevance for the treatment of eating disorders.

Significant future research remains to be conducted before we will understand how yoga influences eating disorders. Nevertheless, we have found a growing body of research strongly suggesting that yoga may be helpful for people with eating disorders.

Yoga and Eating Disorder Symptoms

A common method of gauging the efficacy of a treatment modality is to measure its impact on the study participants' symptoms. If the results indicate a significant decrease in symptom behavior, one might consider the intervention to be therapeutically effective.

To explore a causal relationship between yoga and eating disorder symptomatology, researchers designed a randomized controlled clinical trial of yoga in the treatment of eating disorders.[8] The study included 50 females and three males, aged 11 through 21, with diagnoses of anorexia nervosa (AN), bulimia nervosa (BN), and eating disorders not otherwise specified (ED-NOS).[9] The trial assigned 27 patients to standard care alone. The other 26 patients received standard care, and also participated in 60-minute Viniyoga sessions, twice a week, for eight weeks. Viniyoga uses movement, breath, sound, chanting, meditation, personal ritual and study of texts. Investigators measured eating disorder symptomatology using the Eating Disorders Examination,[10] which includes questions about food restriction, eating concern, weight concern, and shape concern.

Data was collected at three different time points: pre-intervention, post-intervention (nine weeks after the trial began) and one month after the intervention ended (12 weeks after the trial began). Both groups demonstrated significant decreases in eating disorder symptoms from baseline to nine weeks. However, at 12 weeks, the yoga group continued to show a reduction in symptoms, while the control group reported an *increase* in symptoms.

Analyses also indicated significantly reduced food preoccupation after each yoga session. Participants reported that yoga positively benefited them, making statements such as: "This is the only hour in my week when I don't think about my weight."

Another randomized controlled trial of a hatha yoga intervention for women between the ages of 25 and 65 with self-reported binge-eating disorders also showed significant decreases in symptomatology.[11] The sample consisted of a yoga group (n = 34) and wait-list control group (n = 37). All of the participants scored higher than 20 on the Binge Eating Scale[12] and had a Body Mass Index greater than 25. The hatha yoga program consisted of asana (postures), pranayama (breath work) and dharana (concentrative meditation, including instruction in mindful eating). Data on binge-eating behavior was collected before exposure to the intervention and after 12 weeks of weekly yoga. Researchers found significant decreases in binge-eating symptoms compared to pre-intervention levels and the results were sustained after 3 months. The control group, however, did not improve significantly on any measures.

Similar findings were observed in a small, uncontrolled study of five experienced female yoga practitioners with a self-reported history of eating disorders.[13] After participating in a six-day multiple component workshop that included Forrest Yoga (sustained holding of poses, core abdominal work and long pose sequences), the women reported statistically significant increases in body and emotional awareness, findings that persisted when researchers followed up a month later. In particular, women reported an increased capacity to accurately identify, comprehend and respond to their emotional states. The workshop also provided healthy eating training, elements of positive psychology, emphasis on the healing ability of nature and process work. While the women were not formally diagnosed with an eating disorder, they scored in the clinically significant range for symptomatology on a validated eating disorder measure.

This study is interesting in its finding that an intensive six-day yoga workshop improved body and emotional awareness among women who had already been practicing yoga an average of two years, and who "described yoga as something they had incorporated in other areas of their life."[14]

Several cross-sectional studies examined the relationship between yoga practice and eating disorder symptoms. A 2005 study[15] investigated disordered eating attitudes among female yoga practitioners (n = 43), female aerobic exercisers (n = 45) and a control group of sedentary females (n = 51). To measure eating disorder symptomatology, the study utilized the Eating Attitudes Test.[16] Research analyses revealed significantly lower disordered eating attitudes among participants in the yoga group when compared to the aerobics group, and no differences in disordered eating attitudes between control group and yoga group.

In 2008, other researchers studied 571 female exercisers who participated in cardio-based workouts or yoga-based fitness classes.[17] The study demonstrated a significant relationship between engagement in cardio exercises and disordered eating symptomatology, whereas no relationship was observed between yoga participation and disordered eating behavior. The researchers theorize this may be attributable to less time spent on yoga participation in comparison to participants in the 2005 study we discussed above.

The findings of this study support the theory that yoga in the fitness setting may buffer against risk or maintenance factors for eating disorders when compared to cardio-based workouts. Although not conducted with an eating disorder population, a major strength of this study is the comparatively large number of subjects. In addition, the results may be affected by self-selection issues; women with healthier body images might be more likely to take yoga classes and less likely to subject themselves to exhausting workouts.

To date, the findings on the efficacy of yoga in treating eating disorder symptomatology are mixed, perhaps due to the high variability of treatment designs (e.g. length, frequency, yoga style) and the measures used to test eating disorder symptoms. Further research is necessary to replicate the existing findings and assess the direct impact of yoga on eating disorder symptoms.

Still, as a complementary treatment for eating disorders, yoga has the potential to mitigate symptoms of eating pathology. When in the throes of a compulsive cycle of food obsessions and/or negative self-perception, people with eating disorders can use yoga to respond in non-symptomatic ways. Yoga provides a mechanism to reconnect with one's body, and be a witness to the thoughts and emotions that subsequently affect one's behaviors.

Body and Emotional Awareness and Responsiveness

Interoceptive (body) awareness refers to the extent to which an individual can accurately identify their internal sensations, such as hunger or a specific emotion.

Research indicates eating disorder patients commonly experience difficulties in the accurate identification and interpretation of these internal sensations.[18] For example, someone with bulimia nervosa may confuse the physiological sensations associated with difficult emotion (e.g., sadness, rejection, fear) with hunger, and subsequently engage in binge-eating behavior.

Mind-body practices such as yoga cultivate a non-judgmental, present-moment, embodied awareness. Such practices may be particularly helpful if they could be shown to improve interoception for people with eating disorders. Research examining the relationship of yoga to body and emotional awareness has generally found beneficial outcomes. However, the many limitations of the studies conducted to date qualify their results—for example, over-reliance on cross-sectional designs; few participants; lack of racial, ethnic and gender diversity; and few studies conducted with eating disorder patients.

The 2005 study discussed above[19] found higher levels of body awareness and responsiveness among yoga practitioners when compared to aerobic fitness exercisers and women who practiced neither yoga nor aerobics.

Researchers have also tested whether different levels of body awareness among women were related to the degree to which the mind-body connection is emphasized in different styles of yoga classes.[20] In the overall sample, increased yoga experience was related to higher body awareness. Study results indicated that classes in yoga traditions ranked higher in "mind" attributes (meditation, breathing, mindfulness and chanting) were associated with greater body awareness than the classes that have greater emphasis on postures and fitness.

While these findings are intriguing, their implications for individuals with eating disorders are limited. We admire the researchers' effort to classify yoga types and target the question of how different yoga styles influence a practitioner's body awareness and body dissatisfaction (see below). However, the nature of most yoga classes depends in large part on the instructor and the researchers' classifications are somewhat arbitrary.

Other factors may also predict different levels of body awareness among yoga practitioners. For example, might yoga help women increase body awareness even if their initial reason for practicing was primarily for physical or appearance-related reasons, rather than psycho-spiritual ones? Researchers examined this question in a study of 157 women, and found that there were no statistically significant differences between groups; participants in both groups reported body awareness-related benefits from practicing yoga.[21]

In addition to filling out surveys, participants described how yoga influenced their relationship to their bodies:

- *"Before I found the practice, my body seemed more like a foreign space that I lived in. Now I see my body as a tool, home"*
- *"My ability to read the physical signals of my body [has changed]"*
- *"I have better awareness of the connection between mind and body"*

Participants also shared that yoga increased their awareness of feelings that arose as sensations in the body. This encouraged them to work with, rather than avoid, their emotions.

The effects of yoga practice on body awareness were also examined in a study (without a control group for comparison) of 23 predominantly female yoga practitioners participating in a two-month Anusara yoga immersion comprised of six weekend workshops.[22] Practitioners who reported practicing yoga more frequently during the study reported higher levels of body awareness and lower levels of self-objectification.

This is an indication that regardless of the initial reason for engaging in yoga practice, yoga may help individuals with eating disorders gain greater body awareness and body–mind connection.

Increases in body awareness were also observed among 37 predominantly female participants following participation in a five-day, residential Integrative Weight Loss Program that included classes in Kripalu yoga.[23] Participants sustained their improvements in body awareness three months following completion. The yoga classes in this study used gentle to moderate yoga postures and emphasized mindfulness, self-compassion and breathing. The program also included other components extraneous to yoga, such as content related to non-dieting, mindful eating, holistic nutrition, conscious fitness and goal-setting.

All of these studies include factors limiting our ability to generalize the research results: few participants, no control group and/or non-yoga components that might independently account for the beneficial results. Despite their limitations, the findings generally align with the results from two intervention studies among college women reporting body image dissatisfaction.

The first study was a dissertation and must be interpreted with caution, since its results were not published in a peer-reviewed journal.[24] The student researcher randomly assigned 32 women with body image dissatisfaction to a yoga intervention. Thirteen women participated in a 60-minute yoga class three times per week for 10 weeks. The other 19 were put in a "wait-list" control group, and received the yoga intervention after the study was completed.

Most study participants already had some yoga experience. The classes incorporated breath and body awareness, emphasizing the importance of listening to and honoring the body. Instructors used Hatha yoga based on Yogafit, described as a vinyasa flow. When interviewed after the classes, the yoga group participants reported significant improvements in the domains of awareness, the mind-body connection and mindfulness of the self.

The second study explored yoga's impact on alexithymia (the inability to recognize emotions and their subtleties and textures), which is common among people with eating disorders.[25]

The researchers randomly assigned 93 women to participate in one of three groups:

- An Integral yoga intervention ($n = 33$)
- A dissonance-based intervention in which participants were asked to take a stance against the cultural thin ideal through verbal, written and behavioral exercises. Previous research showed this activity to reduce adherence to the thin-ideal and related eating disorder symptomatology ($n = 30$)
- A control group that received no treatment ($n = 30$)

The interventions met for 45-minute classes once a week for six weeks. When compared to the dissonance-based intervention and control group, the yoga-only group had no significant improvement in emotional awareness. These findings are noteworthy because researchers studied a comparison group which controlled for group support and interaction factors that may explain the beneficial effects observed in other yoga studies. This particular group was a very strict control, since dissonance-based interventions have been empirically validated in the mitigation of eating disorder pathology. While it may be difficult for any yoga intervention to outperform the dissonance-based intervention, the lack of improvement relative to the no-treatment control suggests that once-weekly yoga may be insufficient to address alexithymia.

This study is scientifically rigorous, given its three-armed design, and its comparison of yoga to an established eating disorder treatment tool. At the same time, the findings must be interpreted with caution, because yoga's effects on eating disorder symptomatology may be dose dependent. For example, practicing yoga three to four times a week may reduce symptoms or increase prevention to an extent that may rival once-weekly psychological interventions. In addition, yoga may effectively complement psychotherapy interventions, due to increases in mind-body awareness and overall physical and mental well-being. Finally, the results of any one study should not be viewed as conclusive. Multiple studies targeting the same research question are necessary in order to determine conclusively whether a causal relationship exists between X intervention and Y outcome.

Self-objectification

Several studies show a relationship between yoga practice and reduced levels of self-objectification. In the previously mentioned 2005 study,[26] higher levels of body awareness and body responsiveness appeared to account for less self-objectification among yoga practitioners, but not among aerobics users and women who did not practice yoga or aerobics.

Since data was collected at just one time point, we can only *hypothesize* that yoga causes higher levels of body awareness in practitioners, which in turn lowers levels of self-objectification (a proven correlate of eating disorders).

These findings are intriguing when considering the 2008 investigation of 571 female exercisers.[27] The women practicing yoga were more likely to exercise primarily for health and fitness reasons and they reported lower levels of self-objectification. However, participants in cardio-based workouts were more likely to endorse exercise motivation for appearance-related reasons such as weight loss—and more likely to report self-objectification, poor body image and disordered eating. The researchers found that motivation to exercise for appearance-related reasons statistically explained the strong relationship observed between cardio workouts and poor body image and disordered eating.

In the Anusara yoga immersion study,[28] practitioners reported less self-objectification after participating in a two-month program. However, these findings were only partially replicated in a much smaller study examining state (short-term) and trait (longer-term) levels of self-objectification in a sample of eight adolescent females participating in six weekly Kundalini yoga classes.[29] The girls demonstrated a 40 percent drop in state self-objectification after the first yoga session and demonstrated lower state self-objectification after participation in subsequent yoga sessions. However, there were no enduring changes in trait self-objectification observed after the yoga program.

The researchers suggest that yoga may be more suited to changing state self-objectification because it encourages attentiveness to internal sensations rather than external appearance. The lack of improvement in trait self-objectification may be attributable to the very small number of participants, or to the possibility that yoga's effects on self-objectification are relatively short-term. Nevertheless, the distinct possibility remains that consistent yoga practice over a long period of time may reduce trait self-objectification. No research to date has examined this question, or the effects different types of yoga may have on self-objectification.

In the dissertation study of college women with high body dissatisfaction, the researchers screened for changes in *trait* self-objectification following yoga practice. They observed no statistically significant differences between the yoga participation group and the non-yoga control group. Nevertheless, participant reports suggested that some did benefit from increased mind-body connection:

- *"[Yoga] has given me ... the gift of being able to have a conversation with my body. A voice that has been mute for years is finally able to speak and tell me what it needs ... The experience has been extremely helpful in bringing awareness to what my body needs and communicates to me by doing yoga. The conversations between my body and my mind are something I will be able to use my entire life."*
- *"Today I did not spend much extra time worrying about how I looked ... right now I feel very comfortable in my body."*[30]

The relationship of yoga practice to self-objectification is unclear from the described research. Future research should consider examining self-objectification over a longer duration (e.g., six months to a year) to see if longer-term practice is associated with trait shifts in eating disorder patients, and in the general population. In addition, it is important to consider the type of yoga being practiced and whether it may exacerbate, rather than attenuate, self-objectification among people with eating disorders.

Yoga and the Self

Within the context of healthy development, yoga and eating disorders researchers theorize that the version of one's self presented to the external world, or the *representational self*, is aligned with the authentic, *real* self.[31] The theory posits that, ideally, there is attunement between one's self-system (physiological, emotional, and cognitive "selves") and one's cultural or external system (family, community, and cultural influences). However individuals with eating disorders are often mis-attuned. They perceive their physiological, emotional, and/or cognitive self to be unacceptable to the external system (family and/or community), and thus they create an incongruent or artificially attuned identity that suppresses their Authentic Self.

Yoga strives for attunement by promoting a sense of identity that incorporates, honors and celebrates the subjective experience of embodiment in the present moment. At the same time, yoga instructs that one's authentic, true, or core self transcends the immediate experience of embodiment. Yoga employs a multi-faceted model of the self (or identity) which integrates physical (Anamayakosha), breath (Pranamayakosha), mental/emotional (Manomayakosha), intuitive (Vijnanamayakosha) and spiritual (Anandamayakosha) constituents.

In this section, we summarize research suggesting that yoga affects variables that loosely coincide with each of these domains—variables also related to eating disorders.

Body dissatisfaction

One of the most consistent factors influencing the initiation and maintenance of eating disorders is discrepancy between a person's actual body size/shape and how they perceive their body size/shape.[32]

Only two studies have examined the effects of yoga alone on body image dissatisfaction. The dissertation study mentioned above found that, following yoga participation, levels of body image dissatisfaction went down and body satisfaction went up. In contrast, the alexithymia study observed yoga to have no impact on body dissatisfaction.[33] While this may be attributable to the study's comparatively low dose of yoga, the authors theorize that a yoga intervention more specifically targeted to body satisfaction or other eating disorder-related variables may foster more robust results.

Other studies show similar results. For instance, a large, population-based study of young adults found that both boys and girls practicing yoga and Pilates were less likely to report body dissatisfaction than girls who did not practice.[34] A non-controlled study examined the effects of a yoga-based, multi-faceted treatment program on aspects of symptomatology among 24 female eating disorder patients.[35] Researchers observed decreases in body dissatisfaction post-program.

Decreases in body dissatisfaction and drive for thinness were also observed in two studies that examined the effects of multi-faceted curricula targeted at eating disorder prevention in fifth-grade females.

The 2006 study[36] investigated the effects of the curricula among 45 girls and did not have a control group. The 2008 study[37] compared the same yoga curricula ($n = 75$) to a wait-list control group ($n = 69$). These studies, while encouraging, are multi-faceted, making it difficult to determine the nature of yoga's specific contribution(s) to the decrease in body dissatisfaction.

Drive for thinness

Drive for thinness can subsume the eating disorder patient's identity, taking on an urgency that supersedes other needs. Theoretically, yoga's emphasis on the holistic, embodied, subjective self should combat self-objectification and the related desire to be thin. However, comparatively little research has examined yoga's relation to, or effect on, the drive for thinness. Most relevant studies examine multi-faceted curricula that integrate yoga with other elements, such as nutrition education and media education and feminist analysis to raise awareness of the sociocultural contributors to eating disorders. All but one of these studies[38] suggests yoga may be part of a successful strategy to reduce the drive for thinness, but do not infer yoga's causality due to the many other components included in the interventions.

Self-Compassion

Self-compassion acknowledges that one's shortcomings are part of the larger human experience and emphasizes the importance of expressing self-kindness when confronted with perceived failures. This represents a form of unconditional acceptance, and has thus been theorized to foster an increased sense of self-worth and attenuated self-evaluation that helps people transcend situational challenges.[39]

Self-compassion and intrinsic motivation are both characterized by an unconditional expression of self-worth. Intrinsic motivation includes behaviors driven by internal, rather than external, rewards. In contrast, extrinsic motivation is often characterized by feelings that one must produce a skill or behavior to keep self-worth.[40] It is related to fears and/or contingencies placed on a person's sense of their value, and common among people with eating disorders.

Given that many eating disorder patients report an antagonistic and conflicted relationship with their bodies and themselves, self-compassion may be a particularly salient benefit of yoga as an adjunct to psychotherapy. An important goal of yoga is to practice self-care and self-attunement while moving through the formal poses. This helps build these skills in a safe/low-stress/nurturing environment. The practice can then often transfer to other aspects of the practitioner's life.

Following participation in multi-component yoga-based interventions, self-compassion has been shown to increase.[41,42] An increasing body of research has explored relations between self-compassion and mental health in clinical as well as non-clinical populations. However, no studies to date have examined the specific impact of yoga on self-compassion in eating disorder patients.

Nevertheless, there is some evidence indicating beneficial linkages between self-compassion and factors related to eating disorders. For instance, self-compassion has been related in cross-sectional research to lower body dissatisfaction and drive for thinness;[43,44] weight concerns and body preoccupation;[45] social physique anxiety (experienced when perceiving and evaluating one's body);[46] objectified body consciousness; body surveillance (viewing one's body as an object and monitoring it regularly) and body shame.[47]

Canadian studies have found that higher self-compassion levels prior to eating disorder treatment predict better longer-term treatment outcomes,[48] and that early increases in self-compassion while in eating disorder treatment predict longer-term reduction of eating disorder symptomatology.[49]

A cross-sectional study of 252 female exercisers examined the relationship between self-compassion and motivation to exercise.[50] Researchers found that self-compassion was positively correlated with intrinsic motivation for exercise, i.e., a beneficial form of motivation "initiated and regulated through choice as an expression of oneself."

Given the identity concerns of many eating disorder clients, self-compassion may prompt increases in intrinsic motivation for healthier behaviors and a desire for self-care. Self-compassion encourages unconditional self-acceptance regardless of appearance, performance, or interpersonal evaluation—a healthy alternative to contingencies placed on self-worth by the eating disorder. In addition, self-compassion should be more likely to enhance connection with the authentic self. Self-compassion, self-acceptance and connection to the authentic self are central elements of yoga, thus it would seem that yoga could meet important needs in eating disorders recovery.

Mindfulness

A compelling array of research evidence suggests that mindfulness-based treatments effectively address psychological and physical health conditions, from anxiety and depression[51] to obesity and eating disorders.[52,53] Defined as "paying attention in a particular way; on purpose, in the present moment, and non-judgmentally,"[54] mindfulness is an ancient concept central to both yoga and eating disorders treatment.

Eating disorder patients tend to engage in frequent self-judgment, coupled with strong identification, or fusion, with the content of their thoughts. For example, the thought "I am fat" often reflects the eating disordered individual's perception of self-worth or status, rather than a conditioned response to a particular contextual trigger, such as clothing fitting too tightly or eating too much of a perceived forbidden food.

"Don't believe everything you think" is another way to express this concept. When maladaptive, unkind, or harsh thoughts arise, mindfulness training helps individuals recognize such thoughts as thoughts, but not necessarily to identify with them, or believe that they are true. Mindfulness training encourages us to realize that it is the identification with unkind thoughts that engenders distress and negative feelings, rather than the thoughts themselves. For example, believing that "I am fat" may trigger feelings of shame, unworthiness, and unlovability, whereas recognizing that this belief is a previously learned or internalized story that has no bearing or reflection on one's intrinsic self-worth may yield considerably less distress.

Mindfulness is also thought to increase awareness of the relationship between habitual thoughts and behaviors, which in turn may help lead to changes in these behaviors.[55]

A number of cross-sectional studies link yoga participation to higher levels of mindfulness,[56] while yoga training has been found to increase mindfulness.[57,58,59] To date some mindfulness-based interventions have shown promise in the treatment of binge eating disorder, bulimia nervosa, and anorexia nervosa, although much of the research lacks control groups and must thus be interpreted with caution.

In cross-sectional research, dispositional (i.e., trait) mindfulness has been related to lower levels of binge eating,[60] eating-related disinhibition (uncontrolled and emotional eating)[61] and other measures of eating pathology.[62,63]

One important consideration: in yoga traditions, mindfulness and self-compassion are best cultivated in tandem. Reflecting this, in many contemplative traditions, the words "heart" and "mind" are synonymous.[64] Without practicing self-compassion, practicing mindfulness meditation is like "standing in the sun and feeling no heat."

Initially, mindfulness may be most accessible for eating disorder patients who may experience profound difficulties extending compassion towards the self. Starting to observe self-judgment through yoga may help to lessen identification with judgmental thoughts and the requisite suffering. Cultivating non-judgmental awareness of bodily experience throughout the yoga practice can set the stage for expressing kindness towards one's body when it needs rest or care. These embodied, experiential practices may then translate into an individual's self-concept off the mat, lessening the barriers to accessing mindfulness and self-compassion in daily life.

Emotion regulation

Emotional regulation refers to an individual's ability to observe, evaluate, and modify their emotions. The emotional affect regulation model of eating pathology theorizes that symptom use offers distraction from and soothing of difficult emotions.[65] For instance, bingeing can provide temporary emotional distraction and/or soothing in both binge eating disorder and bulimia nervosa.

Despite the paucity of research linking yoga participation to emotion regulation in eating disorder patients, other research allows us to theorize that yoga may be particularly effective. A randomized controlled trial found yoga participation to improve emotion regulation among women with Post-Traumatic Stress Disorder, when compared to a no-treatment control group.[66] A significant literature also suggests that yoga may beneficially affect eating disorder-related comorbidities, including depression[67] and obsessive-compulsive disorder.[68] These findings are supported by the Forrest yoga pilot study,[69] which found significant decreases in general psychological maladjustment and mood disturbance following participation.

Finally, very preliminary evidence provides some support for the theory that yoga practice may beneficially influence affect-related neurotransmitters, which are critical for the regulation of emotions. Imbalances in these brain chemicals may be implicated in eating disorders.[70,71] Research also exists on neurotransmitters that may be impacted by yoga, including gamma-aminobutyric acid,[72] dopamine[73,74] and melatonin.[75,76]

While no research to date has examined yoga's effects on serotonin, all moderate forms of exercise have been related to improvements in serotonin.[77,78]

Spirituality

Psychology defines the construct of spirituality in many ways, for example, proposing that spirituality involves seeking personal authenticity, genuineness, and wholeness.[79] Eating disorders reflect an individual's *hunger* for wholeness. Symptoms of eating pathology have been proposed to reflect a longing to awaken and embrace the whole self. At the core of an eating disorder "is a cry to deepen our understanding of who we really are. It is a longing to know ourselves in mind, body and spirit."[80] The psycho-spiritual approach to understanding eating disorders conceptualizes a process through which an individual navigates various aspects of the Self in an attempt to heal her/his fragmented identity.

Several studies indicate that spiritual beliefs may serve as a protective factor for those at risk for eating disorders.[81,82] Furthermore, research reflects improvements in eating disorder symptoms following spirituality-based interventions.[83]

Although the spiritual aspect of yoga is often glossed over in many of its western forms, yoga is fundamentally a spiritual practice. A number of cross-sectional studies reveal this relationship between yoga and spirituality[84,85,86,87,88] and longitudinal studies suggest that yoga may actually increase spirituality among practitioners.[89,90]

A 2014 study sheds further insight on the relationship of yoga to spirituality over time.[91] Researchers observed that while yoga practitioners and instructors commonly report stress reduction and exercise motives for initiating yoga participation, spirituality was the most commonly cited factor in both groups for maintaining practice longer term.

Although not proof of causality, these findings align with the hypothesis that yoga practice facilitates a spiritual understanding that leads to a more authentic sense of being. The results of the cross-sectional study of 157 yoga practitioners that assessed spiritual beliefs and body satisfaction are also supportive of this.[92] While the inclusion criteria were not limited to those diagnosed with an eating disorder, many participants reported having previous eating disorders and body image issues. The participants who reported practicing yoga for psycho-spiritual reasons stated motivations ranging from "becoming aware of feelings" to "the religio-philosophical foundations of yoga."

In the qualitative portion of the study, researchers asked participants how they perceived spirituality's effect on their eating and body image attitudes, and about their spiritual growth since beginning their yoga practice. Responses included:

- *"Yoga has given me, much like religion does for many of the people in my life, something greater to believe in."*
- *"Without yoga I would be spiritually adrift."*
- *"Before, I was kind of a body walking in the Earth, the mind and body without a spirit. When I fed the body, I just fed my body and I wasn't thinking about anything else. [...] I have an energetic body that I need to take care of, too."*

Given the nature of existing research, it is difficult to discern whether yoga attracts individuals who suffer from poor body image and are more spiritually-inclined, or whether people experience spiritual growth through the practice of yoga, which in turn improves the relationship with self and body. Further research would deepen our understanding of the interplay between these constructs and how yoga could be beneficial to those at risk for eating disorders and those already suffering from them.

Final Considerations

Early evidence suggests yoga appears to have beneficial relations with a broad array of adverse characteristics associated with eating disorders (e.g., self-objectification, body dissatisfaction, emotion dysregulation, body awareness), as well as attributes theorized or shown to be protective against the development of eating disorders (e.g., mindfulness, self-compassion, spirituality). These findings span physical, mental, emotional and spiritual domains, and are consistent with yoga's multidimensional model of the self.

However, little intervention research has been conducted into yoga's specific impact on eating disorders prevention, treatment, or recovery. For instance, we know comparatively little about such basic issues as "dosage," how much yoga is required to obtain beneficial outcomes. This knowledge gap remains even though several large surveys of yoga practitioners suggest that frequency and duration of yoga practice is linked to greater reported physical and mental health benefits.[93]

Future research will have to take into account the heterogeneous nature of eating disorders. The clinical presentations of various eating disorders are similar in some ways and distinct in other, important ways. Drawing from yoga therapy, each diagnosis may require distinct forms of yoga to facilitate optimal treatment.

At the same time, researchers must also address the heterogeneous nature of yoga itself, which encompasses hundreds of lineages and presentations in the US alone.

Many people with eating disorders report that yoga helped them to recover but others may find that certain types of yoga reinforce underlying patterns of experiential avoidance, excessive goal-orientation and the belief that something external can provide all of the answers to "fix" them.[94]

It is important to note that while the field needs better data on the potential of yoga to influence the course of eating disorders, the reviewed evidence suggests eating disorder sensitive yoga does no harm.

In our view, promising preliminary evidence and sufficient theoretical rationale exist to believe yoga may help alleviate aspects of eating disorder symptomatology—a belief supported by the number of patients and clinicians who report it as effective.[95]

Thus considered, yoga's inclusion as a therapeutic adjunct to the treatment of eating disorders warrants strong consideration.

Notes

1 Klein, J. & Cook-Cottone, C.P. (2013) "The effects of yoga on eating disorder symptoms and correlates: a review." *International Journal of Yoga Therapy* 23: 41–50.
2 Beales, D.L. & Dolton, R. (2000) "Eating disordered patients: personality, alexithymia, and implications for primary care." *British Journal of General Practice* 50: 21–26.
3 Pinaquy, S., Chabrol, H., Simon, C., Louvet, J.P. & Barbe, P. (2003) "Emotional eating, alexithymia, and binge-eating disorder in obese women." *Obesity Research* 11(2): 195–201.
4 Fassino, S., Pierò, A., Gramaglia, C. & Abbate-Daga, G. (2004) "Clinical, psychopathological and personality correlates of interoceptive awareness in anorexia nervosa, bulimia nervosa and obesity." *Psychopathology* 4: 168–74.
5 Tylka, T.L. & Hill, M.S. (2004) "Objectification theory as it relates to disordered eating among college women." *Sex Roles* 51 (11–12): 719–30.
6 Garrett, C.J. (1996) "Recovery from Anorexia Nervosa: A Durkheimian interpretation." *Social Science & Medicine* 43(10): 1489–506.
7 Faulds, Richard (2005) *Kripalu Yoga: A Guide to Practice On and Off the Mat* (New York: Bantam Dell).
8 Carei, T.R., Fyfe-Johnson, A.L., Breuner, C.C. & Brown, M.A. (2010) "Randomized controlled clinical trial of yoga in the treatment of eating disorders." *Journal of Adolescent Health* 46: 346–51.
9 In 2013, the "ED-NOS" diagnosis was replaced by the more accurate and comprehensive diagnoses of Binge Eating Disorder (BED) and Other Specified Feeding or Eating Disorder (OSFED). See American Psychiatric Association, *The Diagnostic and Statistical Manual of Mental Disorders, Fifth Edition: DSM-5.* (Arlington, VA: American Psychiatric Publishing, 2013). See also The National Institute of Mental Health: www.nimh.nih.gov/health/topics/eating-disorders/index.shtml (retrieved July 7, 2015).
10 Cooper, Z. & Fairborn, C. (1987) "The eating disorder examination: A semi-structured interview for the assessment of the specific psychopathology of eating disorders." *International Journal of Eating Disorders* 6(1): 1–8.
11 McIver, S., O'Halloran, P. & McGartland, M. (2009). "Yoga as a treatment for binge eating disorder: a preliminary study." *Complementary Therapies in Medicine* 17: 196–202.

12 Gormally, J. (1982) "The assessment of binge eating severity among obese persons." *Addictive Behaviors* 7(1): 47–55. See https://psychology-tools.com/binge-eating-scale/ (retrieved 6/3/2015).

13 Dale, L.P., Mattison, A.M., Greening, K., Galen, G., Neace, W.P. & Matacin, M.L. (2009) "Yoga workshop impacts psychological functioning and mood of women with self-reported history of eating disorders." *Eating Disorders* 17: 422–34.

14 *Ibid.*, p. 432.

15 Daubenmier, J.J. (2005) "The relationship of yoga, body awareness, and body responsiveness to self-objectification and disordered eating." *Psychology of Women Quarterly* 29: 207–19.

16 Garner, D.M. & Garfinkel, P.E. (1979) "The Eating Attitudes Test: An index of the symptoms of anorexia nervosa." *Psychological Medicine* 9(2): 273–79.

17 Prichard, I. & Tiggemann, M. (2008) "Relations among exercise type, self-objectification, and body image in the fitness centre environment: The role of reasons for exercise." *Psychology of Sport and Exercise* 9: 855–66.

18 Jacobi, C., Hayward, C., de Zwaan, M., Kraemer, H.C. & Agras, W.S. (2004) "Coming to terms with risk factors for eating disorders: application of risk terminology and suggestions for a general taxonomy." *Psychological Bulletin* 130(1): 19–65.

19 Daubenmeir, *op. cit.*

20 Delaney, K. & Anthis, K. (2010) "Is women's participation in different types of yoga classes associated with different levels of body awareness and body satisfaction?" *International Journal of Yoga Therapy* 20: 28–37.

21 Dittman, K.A. & Freedman, M.R. (2009) "Body awareness, eating attitudes, and spiritual beliefs of women practicing yoga." *Eating Disorders* 17(4): 273–92.

22 Impett, E.A., Daubenmier, J. & Hirschman, A.L. (2006) "Minding the body: Yoga, embodiment, and well-being." *Sexuality Research & Social Policy* 3(4): 39–48.

23 Braun, T.D., Park, C.L. & Conboy, L.A. (2012) "Psychological well-being, health behaviors, and weight loss among participants in a residential, Kripalu yoga-based weight loss program." *International Journal of Yoga Therapy* 22: 9–22.

24 Clancy, S.E. (2010) The effects of yoga on body dissatisfaction, self-objectification, and mindfulness of the body in college women. Washington State University. http://gradworks.umi.com/34/37/3437155.html (retrieved 5/18/2015).

25 Mitchell, K.S., Mazzeo, S.E., Rausch, S.M. & Cooke, K.L. (2007) "Innovative interventions for disordered eating: Evaluating dissonance-based and yoga interventions." *International Journal of Eating Disorders* 40(2): 120–8.

26 Daubenmier, *op. cit.*

27 Prichard and Tiggemann, *op. cit.*

28 Impett *et al.*, *op. cit.*

29 Shepler, D., Lupfer-Johnson, G. & Rivkin, I.D. (2008) "The effects of yoga on self-objectification." *Psi Chi Journal of Undergraduate Research* 13(4): 168–72.

30 Clancy, *op. cit.*

31 Cook-Cottone, C., Beck, M. & Kane, L. (2008) "Manualized-group treatment of eating disorders: Attunement in mind, body, and relationship (AMBR)." *The Journal for Specialists in Group Work* 33(1): 61–83.

32 Stice, E. & Shaw, H.E. (2002) "Role of body dissatisfaction in the onset and maintenance of eating pathology: a synthesis of research findings." *Journal of Psychosomatic Research* 53(5): 985–93.

33 Mitchell, *et al.*, *op. cit.*

34 Neumark-Sztainer, D., Eisenberg, M.E., Wall, M. & Loth, K.A. (2011) "Yoga and Pilates: Associations with body image and disordered eating behaviors in a

population-based sample of young adults." *International Journal of Eating Disorders* 44(3): 276–80.

35 Cook-Cottone *et al., op. cit.*

36 Scime, M., Cook-Cottone, C., Kane, L. & Watson, T. (2006) "Group prevention of eating disorders with fifth-grade females: impact on body dissatisfaction, drive for thinness, and media influence." *Eating Disorders* 14(2): 143–55.

37 Scime, M. & Cook-Cottone, C. (2008) "Primary prevention of eating disorders: A Constructivist integration of mind and body strategies." *International Journal of Eating Disorders* 41: 134–42.

38 Scime & Cook-Cottone, *op. cit.*

39 Neff, K.D., Hsieh, Y. & Dejitterat, K.A. (2005) "Self-compassion, achievement goals, and coping with academic failure." *Self and Identity* 4: 263–87.

40 Thøgersen-Ntoumani, C. & Ntoumanis, N. (2006) "The role of self-determined motivation to the understanding of exercise-related behaviours, cognitions and physical self-evaluations." *Journal of Sports Sciences* 24(4): 393–404.

41 Braun *et al., op. cit.*

42 Gard, T., Brach, N., Hölzel, B.K., Noggle, J.J., Conboy, L.A. & Lazar, S.W. (2012) "Effects of a yoga-based intervention for young adults on quality of life and perceived stress: The potential mediating roles of mindfulness and self-compassion." *The Journal of Positive Psychology* 7(3): 165–75.

43 Matos, M., Ferreira, C., Duarte, C. & Pinto-Gouveia, J. (2015) "Eating disorders: When social rank perceptions are shaped by early shame experiences." *Psychology and Psychotherapy: Theory, Research and Practice* 88(1): 38–53.

44 Ferreira, C., Pinto-Gouveia, J. & Duarte, C. (2015) "Drive for thinness as a women's strategy to avoid inferiority." *International Journal of Psychology & Psychological Therapy* 13(1): 15–29.

45 Wasylkiw, L., MacKinnon, A.L. & MacLellan, A.M. (2012) "Exploring the link between self-compassion and body image in university women." *Body Image* 9 (2): 236–45.

46 Magnus, C.M.R., Kowalski, K.C. & McHugh, T.-L.F. (2010) "The role of self-compassion in women's self-determined motives to exercise and exercise-related outcomes." *Self and Identity* 9(4): 363–82.

47 Mosewich, A.D., Crocker, P.R.E., Kowalski, K.C. & Delongis, A. (2013) "Applying self-compassion in sport: an intervention with women athletes." *The Journal of Sport & Exercise Psychology* 35(5): 514–24.

48 Kelly, A.C., Carter, J.C., Zuroff, D.C. & Borairi, S. (2013) "Self-compassion and fear of self-compassion interact to predict response to eating disorders treatment: a preliminary investigation." *Psychotherapy Research* 23(3): 252–64.

49 Kelly, A.C., Carter, J.C. & Borairi, S. (2013) "Are improvements in shame and self-compassion early in eating disorders treatment associated with better patient outcomes?" *International Journal of Eating Disorders* 47(1): 54–64.

50 Magnus *et al., op. cit.*

51 Hofmann, S.G., Sawyer, A.T., Witt, A.A. & Oh, D. (2010) "The effect of mindfulness-based therapy on anxiety and depression: A meta-analytic review." *Journal of Consulting and Clinical Psychology* 78(2): 169–83.

52 Godsey, J. (2013) "The role of mindfulness based interventions in the treatment of obesity and eating disorders: an integrative review." *Complementary Therapies in Medicine* 8(4): 430–9.

53 Wanden-Berghe, R.G., Sanz-Valero, J. & Wanden-Berghe, C. (2011) "The application of mindfulness to eating disorders treatment: a systematic review." *Eating Disorders* 19(1): 34–48.

54 Kabat-Zinn, Jon (2013) *Full Catastrophe Living: Using the Wisdom of Your Body and Mind to Face Stress, Pain, and Illness* (New York: Bantam).

55 Chatzisarantis, N.L.D. & Hagger, M.S. (2007) "Mindfulness and the intention-behavior relationship within the theory of planned behavior." *Personality & Social Psychology Bulletin* 33(5): 663–76.
56 E.g., Ross, A., Friedmann, E., Bevans, M. & Thomas, S. (2013) "National survey of yoga practitioners: Mental and physical health benefits." *Complementary Therapies in Medicine* 4: 313–23.
57 Braun et al, *op. cit.*
58 Gard, et al, *op. cit.*
59 Shelov, D.V., Suchday S. & Friedberg, J.P. (2009) "A pilot study measuring the impact of yoga on the trait of mindfulness." *Behavioural and Cognitive Psychotherapy* (5): 595–8.
60 Compare, A., Callus, E. & Grossi, E. (2012) "Mindfulness trait, eating behaviours and body uneasiness: a case-control study of binge eating disorder." *Eating and Weight Disorders* 17(4): 244–51.
61 Lattimore, P., Fisher, N. & Malinowski, P. (2011) "A cross-sectional investigation of trait disinhibition and its association with mindfulness and impulsivity." *Appetite* 56(2): 241–8.
62 Adams, C., McVay, M., Stewart, D. & Vinci, C. (2012) "Mindfulness ameliorates the relationship between weight concerns and smoking behavior in female smokers: A cross-sectional investigation." *Mindfulness* 5(2): 179–85.
63 Butryn, M.L., Juarascio, A., Shaw, J., Kerrigan, S.G., Clark, V., O'Planick, A. & Forman, E.M. (2013) "Mindfulness and its relationship with eating disorders symptomatology in women receiving residential treatment." *Eating Behaviors* 14: 13–16.
64 Santorelli, Saki (1999) *Heal Thy Self: Lessons on Mindfulness in Medicine* (New York: Bell Tower).
65 Polivy, J. & Herman, C.P. (2002) "Causes of eating disorders." *Annual Review of Psychology* 53: 187–213.
66 Dick, A.M., Niles, B.L., Street. A.E., DiMartino, D.M. & Mitchell, K.S. (2014) "Examining mechanisms of change in a yoga intervention for women: the influence of mindfulness, psychological flexibility, and emotion regulation on PTSD symptoms." *Journal of Clinical Psychology* 70(12): 1170–82.
67 *Ibid.*
68 Kirkwood, G., Rampes, H., Tuffrey, V., Richardson, J. & Pilkington, K. (2005) "Yoga for anxiety: a systematic review of the research evidence." *British Journal of Sports Medicine* 39(12): 884–91.
69 Dale, *et al., op. cit.*
70 Jacobi, *et al., op. cit.*
71 Pacchierotti, C., Iapichino, S., Bossini, L., Pieraccini, F. & Castrogiovanni, P. (2001) "Melatonin in psychiatric disorders: a review on the melatonin involvement in psychiatry." *Frontiers in Neuroendocrinology* 22(1): 18–32.
72 Streeter, C.C., Whitfield, T.H., Owen, L., Rein, T., Karri, S.K., Yakhkind, A., … & Jensen, J.E. (2010) "Effects of yoga versus walking on mood, anxiety, and brain GABA levels: a randomized controlled MRS study." *Journal of Alternative and Complementary Medicine* 16(11): 1145–52.
73 Joseph, S., Sridharan, K., Patil, S.K., Kumaria, M.L., Selvamurthy, W., Joseph, N.T., & Nayar, H.S. (1981) "Study of some physiological and biochemical parameters in subjects undergoing yogic training." *The Indian Journal of Medical Research*, 74: 120–4.
74 Kjaer, T.W., Bertelsen, C., Piccini, P., Brooks, D., Alving, J. & Lou, H.C. (2002) "Increased dopamine tone during meditation-induced change of consciousness." *Cognitive Brain Research* 13(2): 255–9.
75 Harinath, K., Malhotra, A.S., Pal, K., Prasad, R., Kumar, R., Kain, T.C., …& Sawhney, R.C. (2004) "Effects of Hatha yoga and Omkar meditation on

cardiorespiratory performance, psychologic profile, and melatonin secretion." *Journal of Alternative and Complementary Medicine* 10(2): 261–8.

76 Tooley, G.A., Armstrong, S.M., Norman, T.R., & Sali, A. (2000) "Acute increases in night-time plasma melatonin levels following a period of meditation." *Biological Psychology* 53(1): 69–78.

77 Sarbadhikari, S.N. & Saha, A.K. (2006) "Moderate exercise and chronic stress produce counteractive effects on different areas of the brain by acting through various neurotransmitter receptor subtypes: A hypothesis." *Theoretical Biology & Medical Modelling* 3(33).

78 Young, S.N. (2007) "How to increase serotonin in the human brain without drugs." *Journal of Psychiatry & Neuroscience* 32: 394–99.

79 Love, P.G. & Talbot, D. (1999) "Defining spiritual development: A missing consideration for student affairs." *National Association of Student Personnel Administrators Journal* 37: 361–75.

80 Normandi, C.E. & Roark, L. (1998) *It's Not about Food: End Your Obsession with Food and Weight* (New York, N.Y: Putnam), p. 119.

81 Homan, K.J. & Boyatzis, C.J. (2010) "The protective role of attachment to God against eating disorder risk factors: Concurrent and prospective evidence." *Eating Disorders* 18: 239–58.

82 Jacobs-Pilipski, M.J., Winzelberg, A., Wilfley, D.E., Bryson, S.W. & Taylor, C.B. (2005) "Spirituality among young women at risk for eating disorders." *Eating Behaviors* 6: 293–300.

83 Richards, S.P., Berrett, M.E., Hardman, R.K. & Eggett, D.L. (2006) "Comparative efficacy of spirituality, cognitive, and emotional support groups for treating eating disorder inpatients." *Eating Disorders* 14: 401–15.

84 Buettner, C., Kroenke, C.H., Phillips, R.S., Davis, R.B., Eisenberg, D.M. & Holmes, M.D. (2006) "Correlates of use of different types of complementary and alternative medicine by breast cancer survivors in the nurses' health study." *Breast Cancer Research and Treatment* 100: 219–27.

85 Hasselle-Newcombe, S. (2005) "Spirituality and 'mystical religion' in contemporary society: a case study of British practitioners of the Iyengar method of yoga." *Journal of Contemporary Religion* 20: 305–22.

86 Lafaille, R. (1997) "An evaluation study on yoga as a healthy life style program." Antwerp, Belgium: The International Institute for Advanced Health Studies. http:// users.skynet.be/IIAHS/publicat_files/yogaarticle120.pdf (retrieved 6/3/2015).

87 Monk-Turner, E. & Turner, C. (2010) "Does yoga shape body, mind and spiritual health and happiness: Differences between yoga practitioners and college students." *International Journal of Yoga* 3: 48–54.

88 Saper, R.B., Eisenberg, D.M., Davis, R.B., Culpepper, L. & Phillips, R.S. (2004) "Prevalence and patterns of adult yoga use in the United States: results of a national survey." *Alternative Therapies in Health and Medicine* 10: 44–49.

89 Bussing, A., Hedstuck, A., Khalsa, S.B.S., Ostermann, T. & Heusser, P. (2012) "Development of specific aspects of spirituality during a 6-month intensive yoga practice." *Evidence-Based Complementary and Alternative Medicine* 2012: e981523.

90 Braun *et al., op. cit.*

91 Park, C.L., Riley, K.E., Bedesin, E. & Stewart, V.M. (2014) "Why practice yoga? Practitioners' motivations for adopting and maintaining yoga practice." *Journal of Health Psychology* 2014 Jul 16. pii: 1359105314541314. [Epub ahead of print].

92 Dittmann & Freedman, *op. cit.*

93 E.g., Kristal, A.R., Littman, A.J., Benitez, D. & White, E. (2005) "Yoga practice is associated with attenuated weight gain in healthy, middle-aged men and women." *Alternative Therapies in Health and Medicine* 11(4): 28–33 and Ross, A., Friedmann, E., Bevans, M. & Thomas, S. (2013) "National survey of yoga

practitioners: Mental and physical health benefits" *Complementary Therapies in Medicine* 4: 313–23.

94 Douglass, L. (2009) "Yoga as an intervention in the treatment of eating disorders: does it help?" *Eating Disorders* 17(2): 126–39.

95 E.g., *ibid.* and Boudette, R. (2006) "Question & answer: yoga in the treatment of disordered eating and body image disturbance: how can the practice of yoga be helpful in recovery from an eating disorder?" *Eating Disorders* 14: 167–70.

7 The Light and the Parasite: An Eating Disorders Story

Joanna O'Neal

I had never done yoga before. But I had heard about it. Supposedly, going to yoga class could make your butt look good. So, I was willing to try it. It was my second day at the Eating Disorder Center of California (EDCC) in Los Angeles. I was 22, in the fifth year of struggling with an all-encompassing eating disorder. Anorexia, type 2, said the psychologist, which meant a refusal to maintain healthy body weight combined with a tendency to binge and purge. I happily accepted this diagnosis, which was far more appealing than being labeled "bulimic." If only I had the wherewithal to be a type 1 anorexic. Now THAT took will power!

My insurance had not approved inpatient treatment, so the day program at EDCC was my current option. Yoga classes, I imagined, were meant to make EDCC more attractive to potential patients in this trendy town. The two previous outpatient programs I entered back home in San Diego weren't hip enough to offer yoga, or effective enough to cure me.

Excitedly walking up stairs to where we would be "practicing," I envisioned the headstands and contortionist poses I would learn, and how great my butt would look doing them. When I entered the small, brightly lit room I saw a man handing out yoga mats.

A male teacher. My heart sank as I thought, "You've got to be kidding." I instantly became skeptical and self-conscious. I immediately suspected his intentions as well as his ability to understand and relate to a group of women. Clearly he was unqualified.

We laid out our mats in a single row along a wall of windows overlooking a vast, green veterans' cemetery. Daniel, our teacher, sat cross legged on a mat in front of us, his knees unable to reach the ground.

"This is ridiculous!" I thought, "How can an inflexible man know anything about yoga? Yoga is where people maneuver their foot behind their head while standing on one leg. Obviously this man knows nothing about being flexible or about yoga!"

Daniel asked if any of us had practiced yoga before. Most hands went up, including mine. I did not want to be thought a novice at anything. We began. In a melodious deep voice, Daniel instructed us to turn our awareness inward and to notice our breath. My mind raced.

As the class proceeded Daniel slowly demonstrated various poses, helping us to find our way into the pose while still paying attention to our breath. Anxiety, skepticism, frustration and hunger all worked together to keep my brain preoccupied. I focused intensely on positioning my body so as to reap the most physical reward possible. I tried to keep up and do every move correctly. But soon the years of abuse and neglect my body had endured became evident.

My thighs quivered in chair pose. Against my will, I had to come out of the pose sooner than anyone else. I was furious. In my mind, this class was just another place for competition. I could not be the first to give up; I had to be the strongest, the smartest, the most flexible, the best.

I nearly fell over trying to balance on one skeletal leg after another in tree pose. My arms burned in Warrior II and came to rest on my bony hips after mere moments. "Listen to your body," Daniel instructed, "rest if you need to." But I was not going to waste this workout by resting!

Soon we moved into the Sun Salutation series, flowing movement that links breath to poses in a patterned dance. My breathing was labored, and I suddenly felt overcome by the weakness and heaviness that was my body. I dropped my knees to the ground and sat back on my heels, with my arms and head resting on the ground in a sloppy version of child's pose.

Ironically, I was familiar with this pose. As a child, I curled up into a ball when I was angry or frustrated; my parents affectionately nicknamed this pose "the snail." Now, the snail was helping to hide my embarrassment for having to drop out while the rest of the class moved on.

I listened to Daniel's instructions and waited to hear him tell me that it was time to get up and rejoin the class. That I MUST get up, because my insurance was paying big bucks for this program, thus this class, and how did I expect to ever get better laying curled up in a ball on the floor? But Daniel's instruction to get up did not come. I tried to muster the strength and will to rise on my own and continue, but my body wouldn't cooperate. I was exhausted not just from the class, but from the years of turmoil my mind and body had endured.

Daniel's voice moved closer, and I was startled to feel his hand lightly touch my lower back, communicating that I could stay right where I was. As his hand lifted I felt pounds of tension release. My body sank into the mat as if it were quicksand. Here with my face on the floor, as the class continued on around me, I noticed. I noticed how disconnected I had become from my own body, how disconnected from my mind and even from the world around me. I realized that I had no idea who I was.

I gave myself permission to stay on the floor. I released my mind's desire to rejoin the rest of the class. Amazingly, I was right where I needed to be. I felt safe. Contained. Supported. My butt might not look any better after this class, and that was okay.

A light dawned on me during that first yoga class. I didn't know exactly what it was, but something left me wanting more. I felt alive, accepted and safe on that mat, more so than I had in many, many years. I realized that my eating disorder, like a parasite, had feasted on my soul. All I had left was a shell, an exoskeleton with no substance and one single purpose: to feed and sustain the eating disorder and its associated behaviors. My entire identity had come to revolve around what I did or didn't eat. The disorder both sustained and drained my life.

My symptoms began at age 17, not long after I was raped by an instructor at my high school. A straight A student who had never done more than hold a boy's hand, I blamed myself for the rape and kept it a secret from everyone. The secrecy and self-blame solidified when I was threatened and stalked by the man who raped me.

Soon, I was internally disconnected from my family and friends. I felt overwhelmingly embarrassed and disappointed in myself. I felt lost and out of control, which I disliked immensely. I was suddenly and painfully aware of and terrified by my body and my sexuality. Some part of me found purpose, control and relief when I began restricting and obsessing over my food.

I was excited to begin my freshman year at a university. After working hard through high school, college was a given, although I did not know exactly what career I wanted. I was living alone for the first time, in the co-ed dorms on campus. I received academic honors my first semester.

However, I was still deeply self-conscious and my eating disorder began feasting on my insecurities. I did not feel right in my body. I often ate no more than an apple a day, and compulsively exercised. For the first time, I made myself throw up in the dorm bathroom. I was keenly aware of males and what I perceived as their sexual intentions.

I lost touch with my internal self and my focus became primarily external. My eating disorder provided relief from thoughts I did not want to have. I began bingeing and purging as often as possible, trying to fill the void that I felt. I ran as many laps around campus as I could before returning to my room and collapsing.

My eating disorder took over my life. I became weak and disconnected from all things positive. I had panic attacks and felt frozen with fear. I was no longer able to concentrate on schoolwork and my grades plummeted alongside my health.

My family noticed the withdrawal, weight loss and new, unusual behaviors. At my mother's insistence, I saw a therapist who specialized in eating disorders. I was very attached to my eating disorder as the emotional "safety net" that kept me from having to process all of my frightening and repressed feelings. It was hard for me to open up and express myself verbally. I liked the therapist, but weekly sessions didn't slow the progress of my illness. My eating disorder was still gaining momentum.

Soon I was seeing a string of psychiatrists. My mother hoped that there would be a drug to cure me. I was prescribed anti-depressants, anti-psychotics, anti-anxiety medication and sedatives. The medications brought a plethora of side effects, but none brought any improvement in my symptoms.

No longer able to function, and academically disqualified from school, I ended up in outpatient treatment programs—where I was a star student. I could describe the psychology of the eating disorder but that did not help me on the battlefield. Each night when the program ended, the eating disorder was back in control.

I no longer had a separate sense of "self" because the eating disorder had taken over my identity. I didn't care to live except to binge and purge. I was underweight, but felt fat, unattractive and worthless. Like a drug addict, I'd lie, steal, do anything to support my eating disorder. I lost any sense of integrity, value and self-worth.

Even though I obsessed over my body, I hated it. I had no vision of the future. I was stuck in my past, my regrets and my perceived failures. But I loved my eating disorder because it was always "there" for me. I could always turn to it to find "relief." Bingeing felt good. Purging felt even better. Nothing else really mattered. After years of daily struggle, I understood that I would die from my eating disorder. I almost accepted my fate.

One day at the end of a particularly bad week, feeling suicidal and lost, I searched on my computer for an inpatient program. I needed respite, if only temporarily. But as bad as things were, my insurance refused to pay for inpatient treatment. Instead, I was accepted into the EDCC, where like all of her programs, owner and clinical director Carolyn Costin had made sure that yoga was an integral part.

After that initial class with Daniel, yoga was the highlight of the program for me. It made "this" treatment different than the others. I began to see myself as separate from my eating disorder. I began to feel "wrong" in my malnourished, abused body. Venturing into yoga didn't stop my symptoms right away, but ideas were planted that slowly took root and arose during my day to day experiences. Strength. Flexibility. Focus. Presence. Breath. Acceptance. Gratitude.

When I first began to practice I felt weak and helpless. It was almost impossible to hold my hands out for Warrior II. My quads burned during chair pose. In downward dog, my heels towered over the ground while my muscles quivered with effort. Nevertheless, my breath began to deepen, my strength improved and the most important part soon followed: the desire to have a strong healthy body, to improve in a healthy way, to heal, to recover.

I knew I wanted recovery but my patterns were so habitual that I was unable to stop. After a few weeks at the EDCC, it was apparent that I needed a higher level of care. Since I had tried day treatment unsuccessfully, my insurance company agreed to cover an admission to Monte Nido, Carolyn's residential program north of L.A. I thrived in this structured environment, where it was much easier to control my symptoms.

I looked forward to, even longed for the yoga classes offered a few times a week at Monte Nido. Yoga helped me learn to breathe through the discomfort that my life had become. Whether I was experiencing a challenging pose or a full stomach, I could deepen my breath and realize that the feeling would pass. I could experience the truth—that the moment or the feeling was only temporary.

My insurance only paid for a month at Monte Nido, not enough to solidify recovery. But I learned valuable tools that would prove instrumental in getting well. Yoga was one key. Another was wisdom from Carolyn Costin. "Just don't throw up," she said. "Some days you will eat a little more, some days maybe a little less, but purging just throws everything off balance." It seems so simple when I write it. While practicing yoga I began to think about balance in a new way and I took in this lesson, which helped me on multiple occasions when I felt I had eaten "too much" and purging seemed "inevitable."

My personal recovery journey took another three years. I had to decide to take the tools that I had been given and apply them. I had to realize that no therapist, yoga teacher, or psychiatrist could make me better. I was the only one who could create my recovery.

Many times I didn't know if I really wanted to be recovered. Recovery was terrifying, even scarier than dying or being sick. It meant having to let go of control and accept all of my faults, flaws, and failings.

But eventually, I was tired of my eating disorder, it was no longer serving me and I was not content being labeled and defined by it. A seed that was planted at the EDCC and watered at Monte Nido was beginning to sprout—that my eating disorder self was not my true self, my dharma, or my purpose.

At one time I had not thought that being recovered was possible, especially for me. I am so happy that I was wrong.

For me, recovery involved these steps:

- Learning to breathe through discomfort.
- Learning to reconnect to my body, one part at a time.
- Realizing that I had a voice and that I mattered.
- Realizing that my eating disorder self was not my true self.
- Realizing that my eating disorder didn't solve any of my problems.
- Realizing that I wanted to live, that there was a future for me despite what I perceived as past "failures."

All of these steps I learned first in yoga and then applied to my recovery and my life. The healing journey is not easy or fun, but it is certainly worthwhile. I don't know if I could have done it without yoga.

On my yoga mat I learned to reconnect to my body, one part at a time. I was grateful when my legs regained strength to support my standing poses and when my arms were strong enough to power a push up. Each asana was like a prescription for earning my body back.

- *Forward bends* calmed my racing mind, quelled anxiety, and gave me the patience to find my breath. I feel safe and contained in my body.

- *Backbends* helped me to bring joy into my life, moving from the past into the present. They help me feel brave and proud enough to face the future and allow myself life and happiness.
- *Twists* helped me "wring out" years of toxic tension and energy my body held. Twists leave me feeling rejuvenated and clean.
- *Inversions* gave me a different perspective, literally changed my outlook on life. They clear my mind (e.g., when I had eating disorder thought patterns).
- *Balance poses* helped me realize how off balance I was physically and mentally. Practicing them motivates me to press forward, to find my connection with the ground and earth. To focus my mind and breath in the moment.
- *Strengthening poses* gave me the desire to be strong and capable in my body. I began to see an underweight body as sickly instead of desirable. I now want to be strong, have muscle, and be capable of doing physical things that I could not do when I was sick.

Through yoga I learned what school never taught me: integrity, compassion (especially toward myself!), endurance, gratitude, forgiveness, respect, love, breath and presence of mind. Balance has to be restored. The practice of yoga is a practice of living in the moment and in all of life's dimensions. Yoga teaches us to be more mindful eaters, more mindful beings.

I am so happy to be FULLY recovered. I have a healthy relationship with food and my body. Eating and body image no longer pervade my every thought. I remind myself to stop and appreciate how free I feel. Yoga has become an integral light in my life offering riches far beyond healing the parasite that was my eating disorder.

Yoga can be adapted to fit any person or situation because its beauty is that it meets you wherever you are and provides you with ways to learn and grow within yourself.

I have profound respect for the practice.

Part 2

Shadow and Risk

8 The Shadow Side of Yoga

Laura M. Dunn

As a long-time yoga practitioner and teacher I know that, if approached rightly, yoga has the potential to transport us from the dim, self-centered lens through which we usually view the world toward a wholly different, expansive and self-aware state of being.

Unfortunately, multitudes of women come to yoga studios seeking firmer thighs, weight loss and a more refined appearance. For those of us who know the destructive impact of eating disorders, Westernized commercial yoga often has a disturbing shadow side that erodes the well-being of our students.

Businesses that capitalize on yoga often create caricatures of what being yogic looks like, and many people naively try to emulate these images through their clothing, what they eat (or don't eat) and even their music. Mixed with commercialism and pop-culture, yoga is often stripped of its intrinsic value, revealing a dangerously dark underbelly. Immersed in yoga's shadow side, students "perform" yoga primarily to master impressive postures, look great in shorts, and feel more valuable in other people's eyes.

The Culture's Lens

Meanwhile, too many "practitioners" misuse extreme diets and fasting as a quick way to lose weight under the pretense of using militaristic self-control to work toward greater spiritual attunement. Lost in these shadows is the reality that genuine yoga practice leads us to become liberated from identification with deeply ingrained, narrow concepts of self; the goal is not a particular body size, shape, or resting heart rate.

It's hard to illuminate yoga's core teachings amid the distractions of celebrity testimonials and juice fasts often associated with yoga in popular culture. However, when we get beyond the surface and the distractions, we find a practice that is free-thinking and anti-attachment. Yoga holds that the realization of self is an inner phenomenon dependent upon our ability to release attachments to external definitions of self which arise out of our entrenchment in familial, religious, cultural and societal standards.

Several trends within modern yoga can snare us into the shadows of self-loathing and self-importance. For instance, a recent issue of a popular yoga magazine promotes yogic austerities on one page, while a barely clothed yogini strikes an impressive pose on the next page. Unfortunately, this juxtaposition conveys the message that looking and performing a certain way signifies the embodiment of yoga and that you can attain this look too with enough discipline and classes.

This perspective fuels the false and dangerous belief that feeling good about who we are depends on looking good and doing awesome things with our bodies. This outlook is a set-up that inevitably leads to feeling poorly about ourselves.

Yoga magazines and commercial studio classes may provide a quick introduction to yoga, but they too often portray yoga completely out of context. We see images of celebrities doing yoga ("to lose that pregnancy weight" or "to look years younger") and we measure our success or failure against their external appearance. The mass media fueled my own youthful self-loathing and distorted my understanding of yoga. The Internet and newsstands only seemed to show images of beautiful men and women in complex and stunning poses.

So, why should any of us care about this phenomenon?

The shadow side of yoga creates challenges for any practitioner—and especially for teachers and treatment providers working with the distorted body focus evident in individuals with eating disorders. Yoga teachers need to cultivate awareness of these conditions, and how an eating or body image disorder can turn yoga into yet another form of external focus and/or need for validation.

My Own Experience with Yoga's Shadow

My adolescence was all about feeling too fat, too pale, too short, or just plain not pretty enough. By age 16, I realized that if I simply didn't eat much, I'd stay thin enough to feel attractive and valuable. By my 20s, I ate so little that I barely had enough energy to make it through college.

Already grappling with issues of body image, eating, perfectionism, and anxiety, I sought out yoga at the local YWCA to ease my body and my mind. The effects were almost instantaneous. People commented on how calm and relaxed I was in the weeks following my first classes.

In the early days of my yoga practice, I felt a genuine connection to my inner-self and developed the beginning of what has become an appreciation for my body. Yoga did what it was meant to do: brought me face to face with my own shadow and an experience of how this newfound calm could be more important than upholding an image of beauty or perfectionism.

Within a year, I became entranced by ashtanga yoga and its promise to "detoxify and purify" the body through a vigorous, challenging and sweat-inducing practice. This was quite a different scene from the YWCA. Most everyone was thin and beautiful, performing feats of physical strength and grace. I was hooked from the first acrobatic sun-salutation.

Blessed with youth and an ambitious temperament, I dedicated myself to daily practice, transfixed by what my body and mind could achieve if I really worked at it. My desire for external attention and validation reawakened as I pushed my body to extremes. I entered the shadow side of yoga.

I quit eating and drinking many things and tried a variety of eating regimens such as raw food-ism, veganism, macrobiotics and other restrictive diets. I fasted regularly and slept little, convinced that this, after all, was what a yogini would do. One teacher even recommended occasional laxatives and enemas to cleanse the colon. A fellow student said he couldn't imagine practicing yoga without the "cleansing" feel of self-induced vomiting each morning. What other people thought became more important than my inner knowing; that had become mysteriously silent.

In its shadow form, my yoga practice imitated modern cultural methods for measuring and valuing a woman's beauty, success and self-worth.

Over the next few years, my old, punitive self returned vengefully, bringing with it the need to control, define and refine my body and environment. Ethical vegetarianism became an unhealthy obsession with food. Animals I once sought to protect I now demonized as impure and disgusting. Little by little, I crossed off foods and activities from my list. I talked to my friends less and less until it really didn't seem like I had many friends.

My partner voiced his concerns repeatedly, while suffering the effects of my self-absorption. I fit all the psychological and behavioral criteria for anorexia nervosa. Ironically, this was precisely when I began *teaching* yoga.

Teaching Yoga in the Cultural Climate

I wasn't the only yoga teacher with an eating disorder history—nor is ashtanga the only yoga practice that can serve to reflect our culture's distorted methods of measuring and valuing one's worth. These dynamics exist in several contemporary styles of yoga. The ubiquity of our Western cultural quest for thinness, youth, and unattainable levels of physical beauty directly affects the climate in which every yoga instructor must teach. We must ask ourselves: How well are we responding to the ever-present incongruity between what we know yoga is, our good intentions and our challenging cultural conditions?

It can be difficult to teach yoga to anyone caught up in the culture's focus on external appearance, and even more difficult if that person has an eating disorder. Teaching yoga brought me directly up against some of my own past and present issues.

How was I to address sticky subjects like food and the body with an anorexic student when I still had body image issues myself? How could I be of service to the development of a student's emotional and psychological well-being when all of my yoga training had been focused on the body, barely scratching the surface of the inner world?

I didn't have many answers at the beginning, but over the years have gained greater awareness.

I am not a certified therapist, counselor, or guru. As a yoga teacher I offer my empathy, acceptance and whatever guidance I can for students who walk through the door. This requires practicing acceptance on a personal level. For example, like most females, I still have an ongoing struggle with my own body image; the difference is that I do not act on these skirmishes. I know that the battle is with my mind, not my body. My struggle helps me find camaraderie with those women who share that struggle alongside me.

I find that offering safety and support to women suffering or recovering from eating disorders often involves admitting my own vulnerability. This admission may or may not come verbally. It may come by acknowledging other people's wounds without attempting to proselytize or preach. I simply allow things to unfold organically over time without expecting a student to be any particular way in class. I try to give people the right to their own humanness. I experience joy working with students on such a deep level—noticing growth and awareness develop over time as each person becomes more of who they really are.

Working in close quarters with people who have eating disorders helped me develop the strength to interact with the often turbulent emotions that arise from the tension between the genuine self and the disordered self, as the sufferer asks: "Who am I?" Of course, this question challenges every human being at some point in life—and is one that every sincere practitioner of yoga asks from the very onset of a real practice.

Our ability to see ourselves as we really are is often clouded by our external focus and a desire for a reality that does not exist in the present moment.

The evidence of my own growth in this process is my ability to see my own impermanence and imperfections objectively and without judgment. I share my own experience of being caught by yoga's shadow, in the hopes that it may spark a discussion and help others.

Yoga as a Spiritual Discipline

Like many spiritual disciplines, yoga spans a continuum that stretches between two drastically different approaches toward self-awareness and self-realization. On one end, yoga brings one toward consciousness and integration of the true self. On the other end, yoga is a method of self-improvement.

Contemporary Western yoga usually lives along the latter end, in part due to the historic dominance of Newtonian, Cartesian, and Aristotelian models of science which hold that only observable, physical phenomenon can reveal truths about nature and reality. Western ethics and religion typically perceive the body and spirit (or matter and mind) as separate and opposing forces, shaping the way we perceive the body and approach working with it.

As a result, Western understanding of self and self-image easily devolves into self-improvement. Society's obsession with thinness reaches far beyond the practical importance of health and wellness to become measures of personal success and virtue. We attempt to manipulate our bodies into "visually appealing" objects that fit our all-or-nothing ideas of perfection.

The Western process of turning the body into a "project" is the faintest imitation of yoga's transformative practice. Classical yoga focuses on the body-mind's intricately woven understanding of physical and nonphysical reality. For example, yoga's concept of "body-mind" is profoundly different than the Western perspective which conceptualizes the body as separate from the mind or spirit.

Key classical yoga tenets embrace body-mind duality to inform teachers and practitioners on how to transform the body-mind along the journey to greater unity and wholeness. Rooted in this integrated and unifying foundation, contemplative yoga nurtures the kind of deep inner transformation which cannot blossom in fitness-first yoga. With practice, contemplative yoga moves us toward an ultimate consciousness and helps us transcend who or what we think we are.

Yoga practices, such as meditation and asana, cultivate greater awareness through one's embodied experience. These states reach well beyond the limits of one's personal physiology and psychology.

It is always important to remember that toxic cultural values and diseased states (like eating disorders) can readily debase yogic practices, using them only as a means toward the achievement of externally defined goals of beauty, success and, of course, thinness.

Yoga Confronts Eating Disorders

Yoga instructors must acknowledge how women teetering on the edge of disordered eating may hasten the slide into a full-blown problem by immersing themselves in yoga environments that promote physical performance and appearance.

When Mary started coming to my ashtanga yoga class; she was professionally successful with little time for much other than career and exercise. Mary attended class religiously, often rushing back to work immediately afterward. She was a petite and thin woman, but neither her weight nor my own struggle with ashtanga yoga's pitfalls prompted me to worry about potential problems with Mary's eating or body image.

We talked regularly before class and she mentioned being lonely since work dominated her whole life. I was glad to see how yoga practice seemed to fill some kind of emotional void for Mary. Time at the yoga studio integrated fitness and a social network into Mary's otherwise busy life.

Within a few short months, Mary had increased her classes at the studio, became a raw-vegan and looked frailer and thinner. She complained about migraines and suffered frequent injuries. At one point, her entire left leg was black and blue. Her body simply did not have what it needed to heal itself, yet she continued to practice despite her frailty and injuries. Like me,

Mary's issues with her body and food must have existed somewhat before yoga, but also like me, practicing ashtanga yoga fueled her problem.

Many of Mary's teachers made attempts to work with her on what we presumed was an eating disorder. We tried reminding her of ashtanga's doctrine of taking one day a week away from practice, and encouraged her to take extra time off when needed. We were even so bold as to inquire if she was still menstruating. Yet I knew any discussion was likely to hit a brick wall if indeed she had anorexia. Unfortunately my negative acknowledgement of Mary's extreme weight loss seemed to be positive acknowledgement to her that her thinness efforts were paying off. My attempts were not helping and sadly, I lost touch with Mary shortly thereafter, so I don't know what happened to her.

Afterward, I made a vow: "I can't make anyone 'get better' but I can first and foremost avoid making anyone worse." I knew I had to make my best effort to embody honesty, transparency and acceptance with all my students. I need to be honest with them about my concerns and accepting of them at the same time. Working with people like Mary might be difficult, but it also offers a catalyst for deeper personal transformation and an opportunity to delve into the wellspring of authentic compassion.

This takes an ongoing practice of self-reflection and self-work. I learned that sometimes it is okay to admit going through my own therapy. This simple act can convey empathy without judgment, and can suggest that it is okay to seek help. Sometimes this is all a yoga teacher can do.

Mary's story raises many questions about how prepared yoga teachers are to interact with students who have or appear to have disordered eating or full-blown eating disorders.

Modern commercial yoga, conducted with the primary aim of cultivating physical transformation, is too often blind to problems like eating disorders that go well beyond the physical. Yoga that lacks the intention of transforming consciousness also produces teachers who embark upon decades of yoga training and apprenticeship without ever working with the human triad of mind-body-emotions.

Rightly practiced yoga has the potential to disentangle us from the confines of a limited self. Yoga helps facilitate dispassionately witnessing our body, mind, and emotions. Through this practice we build a relationship with our observing self. From this perspective we loosen our fractured, and often myopic, associations with our disordered-self, thin-self, abused-self and even our healthy-self in order to integrate these myriad selves into one cohesive whole self.

Letting Go of Yoga to Find It

Elsa was always warm and friendly in my class and had a subtle air of confidence that never once seemed arrogant or insincere. But as time went on, I realized there was much more underneath. She began to make small snide comments about her body. Some were simple complaints about tightness and inflexibility, while others were self-reproaching remarks about her weight. None of it seemed out of the ordinary, because in truth, comments like Elsa's are common among my female students.

Eventually Elsa confided a history of anorexia and bulimia, punctuated by periods of emotional eating. She restricted her diet regularly and occasionally abused laxatives. Sick of "being fat" she had liposuction, only to see the weight come back. She said that her body disgusted her, and as such, she treated her body as a source of pain. She over-exercised to the point of exhaustion and injury. A former athlete, Elsa had a hard time understanding her body as separate from what it could achieve or look like.

At times, yoga eased this pain by temporarily calming her anxiety. More often, however, her yoga experience exacerbated the cycle of self-loathing. Near tears on many occasions, Elsa voiced her frustration with feeling fat and ugly in a room full of thin, muscular women. The competitive, "fitness first" norms of modern yoga continued to influence her practice and cast shadows on her sense of self and hope.

Despite all this, Elsa confided that she had a colorful handwritten sign taped to her full-length mirror at home. It read: "I am beautiful."

Elsa went back and forth between the pull of habituation and the pull of her own wisdom about what was right, often making misguided attempts to find happiness through the power of positive thinking, chakra clearing and other activities uncharacteristic of her keen, rational disposition.

At her request, Elsa and I worked together to help her overcome some of her binge-purge episodes. Among other things, I helped her investigate ways of eating that were both healthy and non-restrictive. We also developed a mindfulness practice to use in conjunction with her asana yoga practice. Eventually, Elsa joined a mindfulness group.

After many failed attempts to change her body by forcing her yoga poses—and even forcing herself to practice when she didn't feel up to it— Elsa finally "let go" of her asana practice and focused on the mindfulness aspect of yoga. She continued healthy eating habits and her weekly mindfulness meditation group. Despite her desires for perfection, Elsa learned to listen to the very real needs of her body and her mind. Her emotional eating slowly settled down as she gave up fasting, colonics, veganism and raw food practices she learned at various yoga studios. Her weight normalized and many of her physical ailments subsided.

Eventually Elsa returned to yoga asanas with the sole intent of being more in tune with her body and her mind. Elsa had to let go of her own yoga practice before she truly found yoga. Whether or not "I am beautiful" is still taped to Elsa's mirror, she embodies beauty more deeply than can be seen in any external reflection.

Enlightening the Shadow Side of Yoga

The yoga community today has a significant challenge: how to assimilate the wholeness of yoga philosophy into modern society without it being reduced by our culture's limited understanding of yoga—and corrupted by harmful values.

Women and men are drawn to yoga for a variety of reasons, including a desire for affirmation and validation. Too often that desire is shaped by a culture that glorifies arbitrary, external and narrow requirements for beauty, desirability and, therefore, value. Any modern yoga environment that validates (or fails to challenge) these cultural standards undermines yogic values—and increases the challenges facing human beings in our culture.

Yoga is a transformative discipline designed to open us to an enlightened wholeness of mind, body and spirit. Yoga is not designed to shape our bodies or feed our egos. Yoga teachers can help by reminding their students that the body is a vehicle to treat with respect and a measure of discipline; it should never govern our lives, dictate our self-esteem, or make us feel worthy or unworthy. Our wisdom and character, our connection with others and with the universe-at-large, are the ultimate measures of our value and humanity.

As human beings, we all need help to perceive our true nature. Genuine yoga practices maintain a timeless quality and light that are applicable to all people, cultures and eras. Yoga must nurture the ability to see within. Both teacher and student must persist to bring the focus of attention back to our inner landscape time and time again. Our real self-image—or, more accurately, our real self-understanding—comes from within, becoming illuminated only when we are silent enough to see and sense ourselves on a deeper level.

Finding productive ways to integrate contemplative practices in the contemporary world is what our yoga—the yoga of modern people—is meant to be.

9 Yoga Teaching, Yoga Therapy and Making Informed Choices

Julie Carmen

Yoga teachers understand the therapeutic benefits of their craft. On its own, however, this understanding does not qualify yoga teachers to be yoga therapists. Luckily yoga has over 2,500 years of history as an effective means for personal transformation. With such rich resources, every yoga teacher, yoga therapist and yoga practitioner can continue their personal self-study, never ceasing to explore the wealth of information available.

In studios or classes, *yoga teachers* usually lead groups of students through postures, sequences, breathing, and/or meditations that help those students learn the rich spectrum of yoga practices.

In clinical settings, *yoga therapists* apply yoga to help alleviate and manage chronic health ailments and conditions.

A growing number of physicians, nurses and other medical professionals are certified yoga teachers, so they can use yoga to address arthritis, bursitis, asthma, joint pain, hypertension, and other health problems.

Meanwhile, many mental health professionals are also certified yoga teachers using yoga for therapeutic ends. Evidence-based trials in mental health journals discuss how yoga helps manage substance abuse, depressive disorders and posttraumatic stress disorder.[1] Academic research continues to explore the efficacy of yoga interventions for personality disorders, mood disorders and eating disorders.

So, how can treatment providers and clients understand the differences between yoga teachers, yoga therapists, physicians and psychotherapists who use yoga in their work?

Yoga Therapists

Yoga therapy in the United States developed during the 1990s in response to the onslaught of issues that our modern commercialized style of crowded group yoga classes cannot address. In one sense, it replicates yoga's origins as one to one teaching and caring for the practitioner.

At present, no government agency or board certifies someone as a "yoga therapist." However, the International Association of Yoga Therapists (IAYT) has developed rigorous standards for reviewing and accrediting yoga therapy schools and their curricula. The course work varies, but always includes specialized training for a wide range of conditions. As I write this, IAYT is creating a similarly rigorous credentialing process to certify individual yoga therapists as well.

The first certified program in a US college was Loyola Marymount University's four-year "Yoga Therapy Rx" program in Los Angeles. It offers four levels of yoga therapy certification through LMU's extension program. Its faculty of experienced (ERYT-500) yoga therapists includes licensed physical therapists, physicians, chiropractors and marriage and family therapists. (Full disclosure: I serve on the program's faculty.)

The first year of LMU's Yoga Therapy Rx trains yoga teachers to work with the musculoskeletal system. The second year focuses on the circulatory, respiratory, digestive, nervous, reproductive and endocrine systems, with additional training in mental health. The third year offers practicum experience with patients in a clinical setting. Finally, LMU's Yoga Therapy Interns spend eight months at the Venice (CA) Family Clinic, seeing chronic pain clients, learning administration systems and participating in weekly integrative medicine staff meetings.

As you can see, three- and four-year yoga therapy certification programs require substantially more depth, breadth and length of training than Registered Yoga Teacher training does.

Yoga therapists support medical professionals; they don't try to "fix" their clients' particular health conditions by replacing psychotherapy or physical therapy with yoga. Instead, they take a detailed health history of the client that helps distinguish ailments within the yoga therapist's scope of competency, training and expertise.

Here is just a sampling of the people with eating disorders whom I've encountered in my work as a yoga therapist:

- A young adult with asthma, scoliosis, a torn meniscus, flat feet, and a history of sexual abuse who uses marijuana frequently and rarely eats.
- An older adult with osteoporosis, breast cancer, menopause, mood swings, cognitive decline, and alcoholism who overeats.
- A highly stressed executive who binges excessively on junk food, and whose doctor insists that he increase his cardiovascular exercise through yoga.

In principle, yoga is self-regulating through its moral and ethical precepts. But as the yoga *therapy* field matures, it is becoming apparent that standards and licensure will continue to follow the evolving needs of multi-disciplinary healthcare settings.

Yoga Teachers

In the United States, most yoga teachers graduate from yoga schools registered with Yoga Alliance, which sets standards for teacher training. A minimum of 200 hours of study is needed to become a registered yoga teacher, or RYT. However, many senior teachers criticize this model as inadequate, arguing that one can barely begin to learn philosophy, psychology, spiritual context, history, anatomy, physiology, medical risks, or legal and ethical parameters of yoga teaching in 200 hours. In response, Yoga Alliance and Yoga-Next (another standard-setting organization) are moving to establish more rigorous training standards.

Since health care, in general, is extremely complex, being under-trained can be problematic for both client and provider. Completing a 200-hour course is a worthy beginning, but it is merely an entry-level certification. Ideally, yoga teachers will earn additional credentials in specialized aspects and applications of yoga. (We see this among the dual- and/or tri-credentialed physicians, physical therapists, occupational therapists, chiropractors, social workers and psychotherapists who are also certified yoga teachers or yoga therapists.)

There is no question that responsible yoga teachers introduce students to concepts about moral and ethical behavior relating to oneself and the world at large. These constitute the first two limbs of yoga and include restraints such as non-violence, non-lying and non-greed.[2] Ultimately, the intention for every yoga professional is to honor the Hippocratic Oath: "First do no harm" and Patanjali's analogous aphorism of Ahimsa, non-hurting. Therefore, it is safe to say that yoga professionals are all trained primarily to care for the student without malice, neglect or abuse.

However, even when a yoga professional's intentions are pure, the public setting of crowded yoga classes and the haphazard practices of the commercialized yoga system can lead to inadvertent errors. Especially when dealing with complex problems like eating disorders (and their frequent co-morbidities), intention cannot compensate for or supersede scope of training.

Eating Disorder Complexity and Yoga Professionals

Properly practiced, yoga is extremely valuable for a person with eating disorders. Nevertheless, the disorders' complexity presents yoga professionals with serious challenges.

For example, many people with eating disorders also have a history of trauma. Even basic yoking (the practice of unifying body, breath, mind and spirit) can be difficult for people whose bodies have been violated or whose minds are full of unprocessed trauma memories. These people often report that sitting still, lying quietly, or being present in one's body actually invites the demons of the past—disturbing the very harmony one hopes to attain through yoga. Therefore, we yoga professionals cannot assume that quiet always equates with peace.

The psychological pitfalls that a student with eating disorders might encounter in a public group yoga class include:

1   Class pacing may be incongruent with the ideal pace for an individual suffering from compulsive exercise addiction or from extreme lethargy associated with depression.
2   Music in class might distract the student's mind away from being present with their breath.
3   A yoga teacher's well-intentioned metaphors, meant to invoke calming, safe spaces such as "a beautiful deserted island," "a lovely open field," "your bed," and even the word "love" may be triggering for a survivor of abuse and trauma.
4   Yoga is often highly effective at disarming layers of protective guarding but this may mean that students return to their busy lives without sufficient psychological containment and closure.

Surveying the inherent complexities of yoga, a student with eating disorders might decide to avoid yoga altogether—or use any one of its precautions as a defense against doing the work of recovery. A student with a troubled past may mistake yoga as the problem, when yoga practices merely reflect the psyche, thus exposing what's going on inside.

In yogic terms, one seeks a fully realized attainment of oneness with the Universe. In terms specific to people with a history of eating disorders, there often are painful obstacles along the path towards oneness. Therefore, these people require dialogue with highly-trained eating disorder professionals (psychologists, dietitians, physicians, etc.) before, after and even *during* yoga.

Ideally, yoga professionals observe and guide students to expand their individual ability to stay calm, present and balanced, even as asanas and breath work become more challenging. There is no doubt that a skilled yoga teacher or yoga therapist, working in partnership with other treatment professionals, can effectively use gradual, consistent application of asana, breath work and meditation techniques to help move eating disorder clients towards healthy integration and recovery.

At the same time, both yoga professionals and clients must recognize that it takes a team of experts providing coordinated care to unravel years of eating disorder issues and patterns. It is unreasonable to expect a yoga teacher or a yoga therapist alone to "fix" the dozens of conditions that can be present.

Implications for Yoga Professionals

Many new yoga teachers graduate from basic teacher training programs and head directly into the belly of the beast: teaching in prisons, juvenile detention camps, residential treatment facilities and cancer wards. In contrast to fields such as psychotherapy, however, few yoga teachers have supervision, such as private weekly meetings where experienced mentors review feelings and challenges that arise when teaching at-risk populations. In fact, there are no current requirements for yoga teacher training to include personal psychotherapy or supervision for the prospective or new teacher. That means there is no process (beyond the competitive hiring mill) to ensure appropriate teachers for appropriate populations.

It takes a seasoned therapist to provide specialized instruction to a wide range of clients with individual needs. As yoga therapist and Phoenix Rising Founder Michael Lee writes: "Teaching a yoga therapist the capacity to adapt the yoga therapy experience to each individual client cannot be reduced to a checklist of instructions."[3]

At the same time, the book you hold in your hands contains the eating disorders experience and wisdom of yoga teachers, yoga therapists, mental health professionals, dietitians, recovered people and others. They are living examples of the valuable education and experience that can be brought from yoga to the treatment of people with eating disorders.

Lack of yoga therapy training does not prevent yoga teachers from becoming and remaining significant treatment resources. Many excellent yoga teachers already possess deep knowledge and experience working with clinical conditions—knowledge and experience gained while collaborating closely with skilled medical, psychological, nutritional, and other providers.

In order for yoga teachers to be responsible and valuable contributors to eating disorders treatment and recovery, they must actively engage in:

- Self-reflection
- Open-minded, consistent collaboration with other treatment professionals
- Life-long learning—which includes learning from students/clients
- Ongoing professional development
- Ongoing personal growth (including personal therapy)

Toward that end, I pose the following questions to help yoga teachers refine a career path that is sustainable because it is in harmony with their true nature and the needs of those they serve:

- Who are you really?
- What is unique about your own life's path that draws you to want to teach?
- Do you prefer intimate conversations with small groups about individual issues, or do you prefer presenting a pre-set curriculum to large groups?
- Are you inherently more introverted or extroverted?
- What populations do you prefer spending time with?
- How have you deepened your sensitivity to this population's specific issues?
- Are you currently licensed in another field (e.g., physical therapy, occupational therapy, or psychotherapy) and are you interested in augmenting your work with yoga methodology?

A Note on Terms

The acronyms after a yoga professional's name can be confusing. For example, both Certified Yoga Teachers and Certified Yoga Therapists can use "CYT" after their names; there's no way to know—without asking—what level of training and expertise a "CYT" has. Fortunately, IAYT is developing a different credential for yoga therapists who meet IAYT standards.

As for yoga teachers, Yoga Alliance Registered Yoga Schools provide the following credentials:

- RYT 200 and RYT 500: Registered Yoga Teacher. The 200 and 500 numbers represent the hours of training completed.
- E-RYT 200: Experienced Registered Yoga Teacher. These are teachers with substantial experience in the field, as well as 200 hours of training.
- ERYT-500: This is the highest level of yoga teacher training; an ERYT-500 is qualified to train other yoga teachers.
- RCYT®: Registered Children's Yoga Teacher.
- RPYT®: Registered Prenatal Yoga Teacher.

Implications for Yoga Students with Eating Disorders

If you are in the midst of an eating disorder crisis, you must do first things first, observing a hierarchy of safety. Seek medical help. (Neither yoga teachers nor yoga therapists are trained to intervene in acute situations.)

Start where you are. You do not need a perfect or clear treatment plan before beginning your recovery journey. Take the first step; if you stumble upon an obstacle, find another way to move in the direction of healing.

If you decide to make yoga part of your recovery, you need yoga professionals who understand the complexities and pitfalls of eating disorders and who understand how to avoid inadvertently adding to the problem. If you already have a favorite yoga teacher, tell her or him about any and all conditions you are struggling with. Ask whether your current teacher specializes in any of these areas, and if she or he can refer you to nearby yoga teachers or yoga therapists who do specialize in the issues you need to address.

I encourage you or a loved one to research yoga therapists and/or yoga teachers. Look online or in person for this basic information:

- The school from which they received Yoga Alliance certification.
- Their Yoga Alliance certification level.
- Whether they completed Yoga Therapy certification with a Yoga Therapy school recognized by the International Association of Yoga Therapists (IAYT).

- Whether they completed specialized training in yoga therapy for people with eating disorders.
- How often they have worked closely with a student or client recovering from an eating disorder.

You can always arrive early to a public yoga class and introduce yourself to the teacher. Here are a few opening prompts that may help a teacher get to know your needs:

- I want you to know that I am in the process of healing from an eating disorder. Is there anything you can advise me about that will help keep me safe during your yoga class(es)?
- Sometimes I get emotional during yoga, so I might lie still for a while and breathe.
- My name is _____ and I just wanted to let you know I prefer to take short rests throughout class. It feels better if I check in with myself to make sure I'm not overworking or pushing too hard. So please excuse me if you see that I'm not always following your directions; it may simply be that I need more restorative practice today.

Once you find a yoga practice in alignment with your overall recovery and healthy lifestyle, add yoga to your list of things you do without questioning, like brushing teeth, making your bed, or washing the dishes. Let it become an activity of daily living. Find appropriate yoga classes near your home or workplace, so you'll be apt to attend regularly.

When you are not in need of acute help, it may be safe to use DVDs or online videos from a reputable yoga teacher or yoga therapist. Home practice with video support is particularly helpful if you are shy or prefer privacy. However, let your home practice be a springboard to building confidence for eventually finding a qualified yoga teacher or yoga therapist who fits your individualized needs. They can quickly recognize common alignment corrections to help keep your body safe.

The most conclusive statement I can make about distinguishing a novice from a seasoned veteran is that finding the right teacher or therapist is (and ought to be) a highly personal process.

Notes

1 See Chapter 4 on PTSD and yoga.
2 See Chapter 3 on Koshas and Chapter 2 on Yamas and Niyamas.
3 Lee, M. (2014) "Yoga therapist education and yoga teacher training: Intention fuels action." *International Journal of Yoga Therapy* 24: 19–22.

10 From Darkness to Light

Nicole Dunas

Consideration of the whole person was something I noticed missing from the myriad treatment centers and hospitals I was shipped to when I was ill with anorexia in the 1990s. It often occurred to me that treating my "condition" as if it could be separated and extricated from me like a bad seed was incongruent with my own life approach. I felt that focusing with such strong intent on the problem helped the problem grow.

I did recover, but spent years tolerating my life and eating healthfully without feeling much relationship to self-love. Through yoga, and my gifted teacher, Sofia Diaz, I was finally able to experience my own form as so endearing, I could hardly believe my good fortune to be alive. For this, I bow to yoga and to Sofia. I have lived without an eating disorder for 16 years.

I now teach yoga to others and have a particular interest in working with the eating disorder population. The following is a summary of my story.

It's 2:00 a.m., springtime, 1995. I've watched food contents disappear into me and then be released back out and into the toilet bowl several times today. With the small shred of me still present to my experience, I witness the fear-based waste of another day. Tears slide down my cheeks and over my swollen parotid glands. The tidal wave of my fear rises so high, it overwhelms my ability to feel the breath in my body that will lead to another breath, and then another, until something, finally, changes.

I see a full bottle of Prozac on the sink. I never wanted to take antidepressants, yet a prominent doctor, in charge of my life in a psychiatric ward, claimed that Prozac might help to un-distort me. Begrudgingly I listened.

By age 22 I have carved words into my skin with safety pins, paper clips and knives, been locked on psychiatric wards, and graduated from a cutting-edge treatment center. I have also managed to pull off a 4.0 GPA. My eating disorder takes precious hours and affords me little sleep; I feel ancient. I swallow the contents of the Prozac bottle. I survive.

Three years later, I am a junior in college living free from formal treatment, and watching my weight oscillate daily due to the intensity of my eating disorder behaviors.

I feel desperate to heal myself through an alternative to the medical system and the kind of professionals who left me feeling soulless and distracted by fear and resistance.

I realize that to survive, I need a community and a setting with routine eating and a lack of easy access to convenience stores or markets. I've been attracted to spiritual practice for as long as I can remember, and have been meditating since I was 16, so I search for a spiritual community. The Mount Madonna Center is a retreat center offering yoga and free room and board in exchange for 40 hours of work a week. The nearest food store is over an hour away.

Facing the unknown, I kneel before the altar I've constructed on a shelf under my bed, and put my head down on the wood. *Great Spirit,* I ask, *Please help.*

The route away from campus traverses low-cut green and beige farmland before snaking up a narrow mud-packed road into the Watsonville Mountains. The black bark of entangled redwood branches darkens the afternoon sun. An hour into the unlit forest, a rectangular sign points me to the Mount Madonna Center entrance. I have not eaten in over 20 hours—a good way to start again at recovery, I figure, since starving tends to calm me.

When I reach the nestled green hamlet, I hide my stash of gummy treats and cigarettes in the glove compartment before entering the low-slung wooden main building. Inside, a tall man with deep-set brown eyes, a shaved head, and a long white beard shows me to my room in the basement.

I was joining the volunteer staff, called karmic yogis; we lived here to serve the center without attachment to the fruits of our labor. At Mount Madonna, selfless service, or karma yoga, is as essential to one's daily life and activity as are the hatha yoga (postural) and jyana yoga (wisdom teaching) classes.

The walls were parchment-colored. Unlike my dorm room, there were no colorful paintings or pictures of friends. The bedspread was monochrome pink cotton. The linoleum floors sparkled with organic cleaner. The lone window supplied a crevice of light near the ceiling. Seeing my new room, I sat on the bed and cried.

On my first day of work, I showed up at 6:00 a.m. to learn an elaborate chai-making process from Sushila Jones, who was a couple of years older than me. She asked me to get 13 spices down from the white wooden shelves. Carefully, I measured each ingredient and set to peeling and mincing ginger. As she worked, Sushila turned and winked. Terrified that she might see the eating disorder lurking behind my yogic aspirations, I gave her a shy smile.

Women who have suffered from an eating disorder often recognize one another. I felt certain that Sushila knew I was trying to end the hell of my anorexia/bulimia by volunteering as a yogi. I worried that she intuited that even as I prayed for recovery, I still felt motivated to lose weight at the center, which locked the kitchen at night.

Sushila did notice that my eating habits were constrained. She tried polite ways to reach me. "Breakfast," she shared one morning, "is the meal that makes your metabolism start running." I smiled. I had heard such attempts at getting me to eat a thousand times. I yearned to explain to Sushila that digesting lunch and dinner in a single day here was an unfathomable improvement. I hungered for her to understand what it meant for me to consider food a material that I could actually ingest.

After my morning kitchen shift, I completed varied tasks. As I made up guest rooms, swept floors, and picked aphids off broccoli in the garden, I was often brought to tears, wondering how I, an honors student, had become reduced to menial labor. Would my parents be ashamed if they knew how I was spending my time?

As weeks passed these simple activities became a relief. I grew a capacity to focus my attention on making a straight lavender-quilted bed regardless of my thoughts or the genuine travesty I viewed my existence to be. Making a bed was a simple series of actions that, when carefully attended to, one after another, were *just that*. In placing my attention on pulling a fitted bed sheet taut, and tucking the top sheet in just so, before drawing the thin bedspread over the top, my mind was released from perseverating on my troubles.

To work without any attachment to what might come of my labor was new, shocking, and freeing. I noticed that I tended to do a better job when I didn't consider what I could gain through my labor. Cleaning toilets with a simple focus on my pattern of scrubbing was a far cry from how I had studied in college: cigarette ashes spilling onto the keyboard as I sucked down a seventh coffee and cried for fear of failure. Without obsessing on accomplishments I hadn't yet achieved, I was free to focus on each piece of lettuce I dried in the kitchen, noticing the leaf's unique shape as I placed it on a towel, folded the towel over, and pressed my hands down to draw out the moisture.

After six weeks at the Mount Madonna Center, I walked into the kitchen at 6:00 a.m., greeted Sushila with a hug, and nearly felt at ease. Each day tasks awaited me. No one discussed the future glory of what we were doing, thus it seemed acceptable to simply do the tasks set before us.

It would be a stretch to say that I was happy, but I learned how to live in a more balanced way than I had ever managed. The yogic focus of placing our attention on what we were doing in the moment gave me a sense of basic acceptance about being alive, and even allowed moments of joy to poke through my awareness.

The Mount Madonna Center sparked the path of awareness that was later ignited through hatha yoga.

Over the years I had become willing to name, and to act on, my love for others, but I had not been able to feel love for myself or my body. In my first yoga class with Sofia Diaz, a physically small, energetically tremendous woman, I was stunned by the brightness in her eyes and the joy on her face.

Standing before her, and receiving her hug after class, I experienced a sense of freedom. She embodied a sense of peace, calm and exuberant light. Whatever yoga this was, I wanted in. I was at her next class.

Sofia took little heed of what I, or any student, could *achieve* at a physical level. Instead, she taught me the ability to notice an experience within my body, *as it was happening,* and how to keep my heart open in the midst of difficulty. I found these skills important to my own recovery and today, as a clinical psychology intern, I teach them to clients with eating disorders.

Before developing these skills, I did not understand that most of what happened in my body was something I experienced through my *thinking.* Yes, if I banged my knee, it hurt; if I binged and purged, I would feel the pain of belly bloat, sore throat and other negative body sensations. Yet, I still had little understanding of the power of feeling the experience of being in a body.

During one particular class, we sat on the floor, our legs long before us with feet flexed and toes spread. Sofia had us raise our arms over our heads. I was in a bad mood. My shoulders ached. I wanted to show up with a feeling of presence, yet I felt resistant to her teaching. I curved my spine a little, to make it easier to hold up my arms. I silently begged her to instruct us to change our position.

She must have noticed my struggle. "If you're challenged in this moment," she said, "call on your greatest understanding of support to hold you up." I tried to feel the energy of the universe running through my bones. An onrush of doubt ran through my mind and a cold, blue feeling entered my heart. I had done this pose many times but each pose is new each time we practice it. In this moment, I was making this pose difficult. What, I asked myself, was challenging on this day about dandasana (staff pose)? I realized that I did not want to feel my experience of being in my body.

Sofia has an uncanny capacity to notice the person who is struggling the most in a yoga class. "Look at your legs!" she nearly shouted. "Notice the exact shape and contour of each leg, as if each leg is the most curious and beautiful form you've ever laid your eyes on!"

I looked down. Big legs. Huge. Fat. I could not even look.

"When you die," Sofia said, "you won't even have a body to express yourself through. Notice the grace of having a body that you can move *at will.*"

As Sofia guided us to breathe down over the surface of our hearts and to draw our breath into our bellies, lighting up our torsos, I uttered a series of questions to myself that were common at this stage of my practice. Why did I show up so diligently to practice yoga? What was the point of keeping our arms in the air and our legs so straight, knees aiming for the mat? How could we benefit from this? I kept up the questions: What if Sofia had no idea what she was talking about?

Through the noise of my internal questions, a deep part of my being wanted to feel this grace, and trusted both Sofia and the yoga she taught as the most important act I was doing with my life.

"If you're wound too tight to feel how you are *absolutely* held in this moment," Sofia went on, "admit that you're afraid. Ask for help." In silence, I admitted I was afraid. I asked for help. *God! I love you! Please help!*

My distracted focus, about what was not good enough about me (my too-big legs, my yoga practice, even my attitude about the posture) made this simple posture painful to practice. My resistance showed up in physical discomfort. Intense bursts of energy pulsing through my deltoids and shoulders felt like they would threaten to take me out. My legs felt sore. I did not want to keep my arms in the air. I questioned my capacity for tolerance and grew yet more desperate. Enlightenment, Sofia has often said, is marked not by your peak experiences, but rather, by how you act at your worst moments.

Not knowing how else to deal with my own resistance, I fantasized about fainting. I envisioned myself collapsing on my mat, Scarlett O'Hara flattened in a flurry of arms and hair. People would rush to me. Rescue me.

Realizing I had found yet one more way to distract myself from being present, I closed my eyes and let my chin drop to my chest. *"Great Spirit,"* I asked, *"Help?"*

Suddenly, the pain in my arms lifted and a buoyant feeling of energy swam through my body. I was still holding my arms up, but using no effort. I felt a presence of bliss pervade me. Had Sofia now asked us to drop our arms, I might not have let them fall.

I could feel every aspect of my limbs in exquisite detail. I could feel the fluid energy running down my legs and feet, the grounded force of my lower torso, the easy lifting of my ribs and heart. How was it that I could feel that good?

Sofia taught me that asana practice is the process of listening to the life force within my body, a process of yoga working through me—rather than me directing a pose to an imagined perfection. She calls it a communication with light.

Experiences like this taught me that the true lack of control I have over my moment-to-moment reality can be as much a relief as a terror. Through daily asana practice, I have come to know happiness regardless of what I am "doing" with my life, or how successful society might deem me to be.

It took time to change my body image perception. For years, I saw myself as socially unworthy due to my weight, which hovered above my pre-eating disorder weight. When one man told me he loved my voluptuous belly, I became nauseous over his desire for what I hated. When another man told me that I had "strong, child-bearing legs," I heard that my legs made me unlovable. I accepted my perception as accurate.

Sofia's energetic insistence that each of us is *always, already loved* helped to crack open my dark ideas and let in shafts of light. She told me: "Be your lower body, Nikki! You MUST learn to BE your lower body!" I would look down. Legs, thighs, yoni (Sanskrit for female genitalia; roughly meaning a source of life or sacred space), knees and feet. How could I *be* my sturdy thighs? Why would I ever *want* to *be* such unlovable parts of myself?

Sofia believed, an intention to change often precedes an actual change. Life is not what we do—it is how we do what we do.

One night before beginning an 80-hour work week at a *Yoga Journal* Conference, I became ill. Paralyzed in fear, I couldn't sleep. I was horrified. I had to start work at 6:00 a.m. I might *fail*.

I drew a hot bath and got inside to soften the intensity of the chills running through me. Looking at my naked body in the bathtub, I felt my usual disgust. But something else became present—a realization that I'd *always* felt gross and disgusted gazing at my own female form. How could I *be* my lower body if I hated my lower body?

I forced myself to keep looking. I noticed the particulars, imagining the moment as Sofia had instructed. Could a new world open to me? Noticing the contours of my body in the bathtub, it struck me that the vision was actually beautiful, immaculately formed and full of life. I continued to look—shocked by my beauty. I began to cry.

Yoga can exacerbate or dismantle an eating disorder. Practicing gymnastic-style yoga asana without sufficient nourishment will beat up the body like any over-exercise. Yoga practiced with an attention on embodiment, care and love can facilitate mind-body connection and healing.

My recovery took huge faith. Some part of me thought it was ridiculous that I could heal. I once told Sofia that I was doomed to live with a "knot like a burl on the Tree of Life" behind my heart. Sofia looked at me without reaction and said, "Get to know the knot. *Feel it like you love it.* Ye of little faith."

The process of healing through yoga is mysterious. For instance, I would practice a downward dog and hate myself one moment, then notice that my spine felt like energized beads of light. Enlivened, I would inhale and enjoy the sensation of expansion in my lungs. Then, I would open my eyes and hate myself again for having fat legs. For a long time moments of positive body-based experience were peppered with dark thoughts.

Eventually, I grew more attracted to the sensations I experienced while practicing yoga, and less interested in the negative self-talk. I would feel a whirl of energy move from my tailbone to the top of my spine and notice that the experience was new, which made me curious. There was so much to learn from paying attention to what was happening in my body.

Noticing what is, as opposed to what I think, is an ongoing process. My thoughts still shape up suffering like an intricate papier-mâché art piece. Sadness might overwhelm me in a moment. Yet my asana practice has taught me the capacity to see my experience as it arises.

Noticing suffering the moment it flares up encourages me to investigate it, which helps me to feel the quality of pain more fully, and thus enacts a shift in my pain. I've recognized my tendency to hang onto suffering, preferring to feel something rather than nothing. However, just noticing my preference for feeling *something*, shifts the feeling!

Dissolving an eating disorder is not an overnight experience. The process involves seeing, feeling and experiencing oneself in a new way.

From the small moments of awareness I experienced at the Mount Madonna Center to embracing my naked body's beauty in a bathtub, every transformation happened in an exquisite pause when something bigger than my thoughts let me relax into feeling.

Now, when I approach my yoga mat in the morning, a calm floods me. I offer gratitude for having carved out time when how well I do matters *less* than *what I feel*. I can surrender to the process of feeling itself, which never ceases to be a vulnerable marvel to me.

For anyone suffering, know that after enough new breaths, there can emerge a new, recovered, authentic you. After enough new breaths, joy founts up, surprising you, illuminating that you are *here*, in this flesh-and-blood life, where experience changes constantly, and where you too, can move from darkness into light.

Part 3

Using Yoga in Eating Disorder Therapy

11 Yoga–Mind Psychotherapy: Integrating Yoga with Psychotherapy for People with Eating and Body Image Disorders

Lori Allen

As a licensed psychologist and certified yoga teacher, I've facilitated Yoga-Mind groups since 2007. Although I am a big proponent of yoga for those with eating disorders I often encounter clients who feel uncomfortable in a "regular yoga class." Their worries are typical for people with eating and body image problems:

- *"I won't go to a yoga class because it makes my eating and body image issues so much worse."*
- *"All I do the whole time is compare myself to everyone else in the room and notice how big my thighs are."*
- *"I am too heavy."*
- *"I am too self-conscious."*
- *"I am too … (fill in the blank with a self-critical adjective)."*

Self-denigrating thoughts and feelings inhabit people with eating and body image issues. They also inhibit such people from reaping the calming and healing benefits of yoga and similar experiences. The constant comparing and self-hatred so often associated with eating disorders lead to social isolation, loneliness and despair.

We already know that coordinated, multi-faceted treatment—especially talk therapy with a group of clients, facilitated by a therapist or therapists—can be a powerful tool for growth, change and recovery for eating disorders and body image dysmorphia.

Elsewhere in this book, you can read emerging research and anecdotal reports supporting the addition of yoga as a mind-body technique useful for eating disorders and related issues.

In this chapter, I'll describe how I integrate yoga directly into both group and individual therapy sessions—an approach I call Yoga-Mind Psychotherapy. It blends the art of yoga and the science of psychotherapy to create balance between heart, mind, and body that can work in any treatment setting.

Why Yoga in Group Therapy?

Although most people don't think of it this way, yoga is, in its essence, therapy for the psyche. Yoga practice uses breath work, self-study, meditation and other techniques to focus and quiet the body and mind. To be a truly healing modality for people with eating and body image issues, a yoga practice needs to come close to the original meaning of yoga: union of body and mind.

Yoga-Mind groups are different from a "regular" yoga class. Yoga-Mind groups are primarily therapy groups; they utilize yoga in a focused, therapeutic approach to help address the complexity of an individual with an eating disorder.

Let's examine the purpose of "traditional" talk-based group therapy to highlight how a Yoga-Mind group differs from a typical yoga class. The power of group psychotherapy is multifaceted, however, three factors emerge as important to the change process needed for recovery from an eating disorder: realizing we are not alone, using relationships to affect our sense of self and providing "corrective emotional experiences."

1. Realizing we are not alone. Despite the complexity of human problems, group therapy shows us that our core insecurities about sense of worth and the ability to relate to others are universal. This experience offers healing by helping to lift shame. For example, we begin to feel empathy and concern for the lovely woman across the room who binges all night after a hard day at work. This experience creates a mirror for self-compassion.

2. Using relationships to affect our sense of self. Since we are a social species, much of personality development is inevitably the product of interaction with other significant human beings. Naturally, we all develop a sense of self that is based, to one degree or another, on our understanding of how others see us.

Negotiating how we value ourselves within relationships is a crucial step to developing a strong sense of self and self-worth. Group therapy provides a safe space to uncover our existing patterns of being in relationship with others—and with our selves. Group therapy allows us to practice assertiveness, ask honest questions of other people, and get feedback about our particular communication and relationship style. We get to know and trust each other as we become contributing members of a healing process.

Rather than residing in our long-held image of ourselves as unworthy, annoying, or over-emotional, we can get direct feedback and experiment with new skills. Our fellow participants help us (and themselves) to decrease rigid thinking with gentle reminders to question mindreading, over-generalizing, or catastrophizing. The practice of being in group therapy helps us challenge seemingly inflexible beliefs about ourselves.

3. Providing "corrective emotional experiences." Psychosomatic medicine pioneer Franz Alexander coined this term and stated that a fundamental aspect of psychological treatment is "to expose the patient, under more

favorable circumstances, to emotional situations that she could not handle in the past."[1]

Group therapy can help facilitate the expression of feelings that may not have been allowed in a person's family of origin. Living in the context of a safe and committed group, members can work through their conflicts and often emerge with more empathy for and understanding of each other.

How can Yoga Contribute to Group Psychotherapy?

For people with eating disorders, group situations (whether a yoga class or a therapy group) often create the sense of feeling vulnerable, overwhelmed, or out of control. These are precisely the feelings that our clients must cope with in healthier ways if they are to recover. Overwhelming feelings can lead someone with an eating disorder into a cycle of binging, restricting, purging, and/or other symptom use. Yoga skills can intervene to disrupt such a cycle.

Bringing yoga into the group format allows participants to release the physical manifestations of their distress in beneficial and healing ways. Integrating yoga with group therapy introduces a variety of new and nourishing practices for coping with difficult feelings. For example, if a client reveals, "I ate a gallon of ice cream last night," this might evoke uncomfortable feelings throughout the group. The facilitator can then lead the group through a series of calming poses. Between each pose, ask clients to notice what happens to their feelings. After a few minutes in poses, individual and group distress usually subsides, and people feel calmer.

Poses can also work as part of the "corrective emotional experience." When we attempt a handstand or fold into a forward bend, we experience the different parts of our body relating to each other in new ways. This is a reminder that we can learn new ways of dealing with challenge and relating to feelings of fear and safety. Yoga introduces new tools to understand physical and emotional experience, bringing these into the therapeutic process.

Integrating mind-body in a group increases the likelihood that clients will translate this practice into real life situations. Yoga-infused group therapy can help bring a person's mind to the here-and-now, and bridge the mind-body dissociation so common in eating disorders.

How to Integrate Yoga in Group Therapy

There are many ways to integrate yoga into a therapy group. Here is the sequence of activities I've used for years, with positive therapeutic results:

- Breathwork/centering
- Check-in
- Psychoeducation theme/topic related to Eating Disorders

- Warm-up asana
- Group work (CBT, DBT, ACT activity, journaling)
- Asana focused on the day's topic (e.g. inversions for calm; heart openers for energy)
- Meditation (specifically oriented to ED issues)
- Savasana (taking time to integrate what we have done and learned)

I begin the group with breath work (such as the basic, conscious breathing known as Ouji or Ujjayi breath) and a simple grounding asana (such as sun salutations). Breathwork can be such a powerful tool that many yogic traditions use it only after asana. However, I find that teaching a light version of yogic breath helps clients to get settled. After grounding activities, the tone and content of group conversation are noticeably different. If given time to settle in and release minor stressors through grounding asanas, client interactions often gravitate to more important, universal themes.

From grounding, we proceed to check-in and introduce the day's theme. People talk about their current issues and describe how they are feeling right now. As the group progresses, members use this time to practice inter-personal skills such as asking direct questions, requesting feedback about interactions, and providing effective support.

After check-in, we do more movement. I usually tailor this asana to the day's theme. The group might do sun-salutations to warm-up and shift attention away from the "distracted thoughts" and into the body and the moment. The asanas stretch and strengthen the body, while also acting as a source of mindfulness meditation.

Using asana as metaphor is a key component to the Yoga-Mind group. Observing through the eyes of yoga, I have fun finding the connection between asanas and the issues arising in a group each day. For example, if the theme is attachment, we use poses to notice when we become attached to an outcome. I ask questions like:

- Are we letting the pose be exactly as it is for us at the moment, or are we pushing and pulling it towards an ideal of perfection?
- Can you let go of expectation right now, and notice exactly what you need to work on in the moment?
- What are some attachments to outcomes that overwhelm you in your everyday life? Losing weight, getting straight As, or saying exactly the right thing?
- Can you imagine letting go of the expectation and coming back into the current moment, just like you are doing in this pose?

These yoga practices help clients (and providers) shift their focus toward the healthy, genuine self. We learn how to recognize the chatter of voices filling our daily life, and hear them without judgment or attachment. We also learn how we can find the voice that brings us back to our breath. This practice helps us identify and attend to our healthy voice and not our eating disorder voice.

After theme-based asana, the group focuses on a psycho-educational component. In my experience, basic knowledge of eating disorder dynamics and current research helps clients gain perspective on (and, ideally, detachment from) the disorder.

In Yoga-Mind group, clear cognitive understanding remains important; for example, teaching clients what promotes recovery (self-care, self-compassion, mindfulness) and what hinders it (dieting, looking at fashion magazines, weighing). As with "traditional" therapy, we use journaling to deepen awareness on cognitive, emotional, spiritual and psychological levels.

I also do group work derived from Acceptance and Commitment Therapy (ACT) and Dialectical Behavioral Therapy (DBT) to help members understand the origins and current function of their eating disordered behavior and help reinforce healthy coping strategies.

Next, we practice poses and sequences, keeping the focus on that day's theme. The following themes emerge regularly in Yoga-Mind Groups:

- The Higher Self (yoga's conception of the Healthy Self)
- Non-attachment
- Relationship between fear and joy
- Being present
- Nourishment
- Intimacy
- Being in our bodies
- Expectations
- Clear communication (verbal and non-verbal)
- Taking yoga into everyday life

Next, group members practice a few minutes of meditation.

Yoga teaches that all minds have tendencies. Someone with anxiety tends toward predicting the worst in a projected future, rather than staying in the present moment. A depressed mind tends to ruminate on past mistakes, without noticing the gifts of the present (like the beautiful Oregon mountains my clients and I see on the horizon every day).

I ask clients to think about chronically distressed minds as under-regulated and under-developed—like the mind of a healthy toddler. The two-year-old child will naturally test boundaries, make demands, and then throw a tantrum if the desired result doesn't materialize. However, it is not healthy for the child to go along in life without mental and emotional boundaries, just as it is not healthy for an adult mind to run unbridled.[2]

Effective parents teach proper mental and emotional regulation to their two-year-olds. Meditation teaches us the discipline of mindfulness. Meditative practices provide a parent-like soothing in response to the mind's tendency to overreact. They focus attention on the senses to counter our clients' tendency to use symptoms when they follow their minds into catastrophic thinking.

Meditation builds up the mind's capacity for strong boundaries that resist mental activity like rumination. It also helps reduce the tendency to attach a transitory feeling to one's ongoing identity (e.g., "I am anxious") by developing our capacity for observing the present without judgment and separating ourselves from the feeling (e.g. "I have anxiety right now"). With practice, we develop the mental tendency to release our attention from past and future worries as we attend to the present moment.

To close the group, we lie back on the mat. We then relax into some floor stretches and finish by shifting into savasana, a supine pose of total relaxation.

Normally savasana is difficult for people with eating disorders; they often state that they do not like lying down and closing their eyes. They frequently experience distress when not busy or distracted due to intrusive thoughts, the belief that they don't deserve total relaxation, and/or urges to constantly be productive or move on to the next thing. Most people with eating disorders feel that their worst fears (e.g., getting fat) will come true, if they stop striving for thinness. Underlying these fears is the fear of not being good enough just as they are.

In contrast, savasana can be used to help overcome fears of relaxing and letting go. A practice of just being, savasana forces us to be in the moment and stop striving. After practicing savasana a few times—with permission to notice the ebb and flow of their anxiety in the pose—clients actually do relax, sometimes for the first time since they can remember. In that moment, they embody self-care and self-love.

Yoga is a discipline designed to address all aspects of human nature. The poses are meant to guide the mind, not to compel the body into physical perfection. We must keep this awareness central when working alongside people with eating disorders, since many of them have used yoga primarily as a form of aerobic exercise.

When people with eating disorders come to a Yoga-Mind group (or participate in a well-balanced yoga class), they learn to focus inward, so that they can hear their healthy, highest selves guiding them into a better life.

Yoga in Individual Therapy Sessions

Yoga was developed, thousands of years ago, to be taught one-on-one in a teacher-student relationship. The two worked together closely with techniques uniquely oriented to the student's particular situation, mental propensities and body type. In other words, yoga's historical practice has more in common with individual therapy than it does with the yoga classes so prevalent in the modern West. Although group classes can teach techniques and philosophy, they don't allow for the high level of transformative attunement possible in one-on-one interactions. Helping clients find techniques that work for their specific issues and physiology is a goal of both yoga and psychotherapy.

Does incorporating yoga into an individual therapy session mean having clients discuss childhood issues while in a handstand? No—the process is much easier than that—for therapist and client alike—as you'll see through a case study and examples.

As veteran eating disorder therapist Carolyn Costin says, "Our job as therapists is to help put the Eating Disorder out of a job." The first step is recognizing that—however they started—restriction, overeating, binging and purging eventually become attempts at emotional regulation. A key treatment goal is for the client to learn healthier, more productive ways to respond to his or her feelings and to live mindfully.

Bringing yoga into the therapy room adds immensely to the repertoire of tools available to help clients understand relationships between their emotions, thoughts and physiology. As neuroscience highlights the powerful impact somatic work can have on the psyche, psychologists have good reason to incorporate the body and breath into their sessions.

I have clients who state they have never explored whether or how much they care about being thin and attractive. Instead, they operate under the conditioned assumption that a certain body shape is, and should be, their desired goal. They have little, if any, experience with tuning into their needs and desires. They often state they don't know when they are hungry, how they feel, or what they want to do.

Asana, breathing, and meditation are more difficult than one might think for people disconnected from their very essence. That's why it can take weeks for clients to become comfortable with internally focused yoga practices. However, once they stop trying to "copy the teacher" and begin to move in response to what their bodies need at the moment, the shift is immediately evident.

How to Use Yoga in Individual Therapy

What does an individual "talk and yoga therapy" session look like?

Over the years, I developed a format that has both structure and freedom to use the relationship and what emerges to guide the session. The format has parallels to my group approach and also seems to help clients relax and feel safe with the combination of traditional therapy and yogic techniques.

Although sessions can be done in an office setting, I do mine in a studio, which invites exploration in a broader space. No matter where you work, you can use easy-to-store yoga essentials like blankets, blocks and mats for support in movement and meditation.

Introspective Awareness

We begin with five minutes on the mat, as the client tunes in to his or her body, emotions and thoughts. Next I ask clients to comment, following the format of typical "check in" questions psychologists ask in a therapy session. Are there areas of physical tightness? Any pain? Areas which are loose and relaxed? What is the state of your mind? Distracted? Agitated? Dull? Is there a prominent emotional state? Anxious? Depressed?

When Casey, a client with severe anorexia, first began the yoga psychotherapy sessions with me, she was completely dissociated from her body. This checking in practice helped her regain awareness of body sensations, thoughts and feelings because I always asked her to articulate specifically what she noticed about herself, e.g. "My hamstrings are very stiff, my neck hurts, my breath is shallow, my mind is agitated and focused on how fat I am."

Because we used the same check in each session, we both noticed the difference in her relationship to herself over time. She began to report more subtle aspects of what was going on in her mind and body, until one day she said, "I am a little bit hungry." This was a huge shift from the early sessions when she was sure her body did not have the capability to inform her about when or how much to eat. Casey's experience introduced her to awareness of the body and the mind—observing them without judgment or attachment—while teaching her to shift attention from thoughts to emotions and breath.

Using Breath

After the check in, we do breath work. Together, we observe how various yogic breathing techniques affect the client's physiological state. For example, a particular technique may soothe one client and spark anxiety in another. By teaching breathing techniques to each client and checking for effects, a depth of self-understanding takes place—moving clients beyond thoughts and into deeper physiological responses.

Breath drives our nervous system and our nervous system drives our breath. If we are conscious of the interrelation between our physiological state and our breath, we can use breathing techniques to steer ourselves in and out of reactive states. Yoga teaches how to make breath the focus of attention, so we can calm the mind when thoughts or feelings seem overwhelming. As breathing techniques calm or excite the nervous system and focus the mind, they provide healthier coping skills and emotional regulation.

My clients are often amazed at how much physiologic change five minutes of breath work can bring. These dramatic and prompt shifts in ruminative thinking and anxious feelings often open the door to a hopefulness that was elusive before. If a client can feel this much change this quickly, she can see that her mind and body must be more flexible than she believed.

Of course, these experiences are fleeting at first and it is important to explain how our work is a joint experiment to show that change is possible. It's also important to encourage and support continued practice; as many yoga practitioners say: "Yoga is 1 percent theory and 99 percent practice."

Talk Therapy

This portion of a Yoga-Mind session looks just like traditional psychotherapy. We assess symptoms, identify themes, notice emotional and cognitive patterns, and decide where to focus. The client and I collaboratively and explicitly choose a focus for intervention or yoga practice. I like to remain in the yoga studio for this part of the session, sitting on mats or chairs, so that the mood is maintained and it's convenient to move to the subsequent activities.

This is a time and space of reflection for the client, who is now more available to her present experience. I also use yoga and psychotherapy techniques to attune myself to the client's emotional state, affect, breathing, self-talk, and issues. The yoga perspective enhances my therapeutic multi-level observing and my emotional mirroring, which can help the client feel seen and heard.

My client Casey came into a session upset that her nutritionist wanted her to add a bagel to her meal plan. Casey stated that she was obsessing about the bagel during the first two portions of our session. We identified the fear-based stories (cognitive distortions) she associated with eating a bagel. We articulated her catastrophizing, black-or-white thinking: "If I eat one, I will become obese. I will never stop eating bagels and carbs." She obviously felt out of control of what or how much she could eat. More importantly, she was taking her thoughts as almighty truths, without any sense of perspective.

In the moments when Casey is dissociated from her body as a result of her obsession with her theoretical bagel, she is experiencing distress similar to if she had already eaten the bagel. She has stepped into her mental tendency to focus all her attention on her fear-based thoughts. She is unaware of her ability to disengage or attend to something else.

We decided together to focus that day's work on these overwhelming and "stuck" thoughts in our therapeutic conversation and the ensuing asana.

Asana

Asana poses and sequences give therapists many ways to combine their theoretical orientation with yoga. For example, asana reiterates and enriches the client's experience with Acceptance and Commitment Therapy metaphors which themselves are concepts also seen in Buddhism.

One such ACT metaphor describes our thoughts and feelings as passengers on a bus. Often, many of the passengers are yelling, screaming that they are scared, insisting that we turn this way or that, etc. We forget that the driver of our bus (i.e., our life) is our healthy self or highest self. The only function of our thoughts and feelings is to inform the driver; they can't actually drive the bus.

When we only listen to the loudest thoughts and feelings, we may forget that we have other passengers—and forget that we have a destination we want to drive toward. When we spend our energy listening to the loudest passengers, we drive in circles or never leave the curb. ACT asks us to reflect on our values and goals so that we have a clear destination—and to remain aware that we (not the passengers) are the drivers of our bus. ACT also reminds us that we are in relationship with our thoughts and feelings; therefore, we can mindfully choose how to utilize them in our daily life.

Asana poses help clients embody the practice of focusing attention on the road and directing the bus toward their goal. For example, certain poses demonstrate experientially that where we focus our attention matters. Tree pose requires standing on one leg and maintaining balance. If we are distracted by objects in the room or negative self-talk, we are much more likely to fall out of the pose. A key to good balance in tree pose is to keep our eyes focused steadily on something straight ahead of us.

Casey tends to over-exercise and struggles to slow down and rest her body and mind. So, we designed a sequence that meets her where she is. It begins with poses requiring exertion, but then moves to slower and quieter poses. I work with every client to create sequences that respond to his or her individual needs.

As we move through the poses I ask Casey to focus her attention. First we attend to her feet, noting how she is standing. Is her weight forward or back? Can she maintain the focus on her feet while we shift into the next pose? I then check in and ask if she was able to sustain attention on the feet. We continue our work in response to her answers. With practice, she is learning to focus her mind and develop a higher level of perspective on the relationship between her body and mind.

As we move into the next pose, I ask her to attend to her breath while moving in and out of poses, keeping the inhale deep and even, and then extending the exhale to the same duration. This dual attending is important in our work because it helps Casey learn to experience a trigger while staying present in the moment. This is very different than becoming consumed by the emotional trigger, with little or no recognition that she is actually safe in the room.

Casey's ability to focus her attention on something other than overwhelming feelings or terror-based thoughts will determine whether she will eat the bagel and/or purge afterward. If, after eating the bagel, she can attend to the fact that she is safe in her house with her dog for the moment, Casey has space to choose where to focus her attention next. We do not try to get rid of feelings or thoughts but rather practice conscious shifts in where she puts her attention in response to the feelings or thoughts.

As she learns poses that quiet the nervous system, she feels and observes the differences in her body. This helps her learn how to use these mindfulness techniques for daily tasks and move toward larger goals, rather than veering off course with internal distractions.

At the end of asana, I ask Casey if she noticed any shifts in her mental patterns. Her face lights up with a sudden recognition. "That is the longest period of time I have not obsessed about food or my body that I can remember." Without struggling, Casey had consciously shifted her attention away from Eating Disorder thoughts. Of course, this short mindfulness moment will not heal her anorexia, but it provides a recovery experience that—with practice—can become a solid part of her recovery toolbox.

Asana can enhance the psychotherapy in dozens of ways. If a client is depressed, we might explore poses that excite the client's nervous system, while we observe the asana's effect on mood. To help learn self-soothing, we might do restorative yoga with blankets over the chest and torso to calm and relax the nervous system, again noticing the effects on thoughts and feelings.

Meditation

Many psychologists use meditation in their practices. I find clients quite receptive to meditation after practicing asana to enhance understanding of the mind-body connection. I teach active and passive meditation, and ask clients to observe which methods help most in quieting their minds. Some people can visualize easily and this helps hold their attention, while others find calmness in allowing the mind to be the observer of thoughts, like sitting on a warm sandy beach watching seagulls fly by.

I teach very short meditations at the start. Five minutes is enough to get most people intrigued by the process and then, over time, we gradually increase the time to 15 minutes.

Savasana

One powerful gift of yoga is teaching our clients the importance of balance between exertion and relaxation. Savasana is the act of integrating what we've just done while intentionally letting go of connection to doing anything. Sounds easy, but it can be one of the most difficult poses!

A lovely and important aspect of savasana is taking time to let things settle. Like the flakes in a snow globe, we allow our muscles to rest and restore after our asana work. When a client has embodied savasana, we have another foundation to teach the equal importance of pausing for self-care and restoration after difficult emotional work like eating the bagel, calling a friend instead of purging, or sitting with difficult feelings.

This allows our nervous system to come back into homeostasis before moving onto the next experience. Savasana can create healing that allows us to bounce back from life stressors and nurture what yoga therapist Sarahjoy Marsh terms our "emotional buoyancy."

Final Check-In

I wrap up individual sessions by having the client recall any aspects of our work that changed or resonated with their mood or physiology. This review reinforces the impact yoga has on the healthy or higher self.

Yoga emphasizes that practice brings transformation. I usually ask each client to develop a regular practice outside of our sessions, beginning with five minutes of stretching followed by five minutes of meditation. When they do this, we both see the development of healing change and on-going mindfulness.

Why It Works

If we are enmeshed with our thoughts, bodies, partners, parents, emotions, or food, we are not living in right relationship with them—or ourselves. People with eating disorders have difficulty with the reality that we are not our thoughts, we are not our emotions, and we are not our bodies.

When we over-identify with anything—our bodies, thoughts, or feelings—we cannot see clearly. However, honest exploration of our relationships with food, thoughts, bodies, and emotions allows for change. Yoga practice and philosophy gently invites us into this inner exploration and provides us with concrete tools that support responding rather than reacting to life's many challenges.

Doing yoga during therapy may feel uncomfortable for therapists who have remained stationary throughout hundreds of sessions. However, as our conceptualization of therapy evolves, our therapeutic techniques also must evolve.

As we learn throughout this book, psychotherapy can incorporate yoga in a variety of ways—and with solid rationale. For example, research on breathing practices, meditation and yoga poses highlights the fact that we have more control over our physiology and neurology than previously thought.

Moving into a specific pose may affect emotional balance by increasing or decreasing levels of stress hormones.[3] Meditation helps increase gray matter in areas of the brain associated with empathy, emotional regulation and complex problem solving.[4] Breath drives our nervous system and can help us move from fight, flight, or freeze states into a calm and clear space.[5]

These practices often help clients create physiological change in very different ways than traditional talk therapy does. Yoga-infused psychotherapy opens the door for exciting new practices, such as teaching yogic breath work at the end of a talk therapy session so an anxious client takes a helpful tool into the week ahead, or developing a more extensive yoga session where a client uses asana to alter physiology and/or explore thoughts and feelings.

As Bessel van der Kolk writes: "Our educational system, as well as many of the methods that profess to treat trauma, tend to bypass this emotional-engagement system and focus instead on recruiting the cognitive capacities of the mind. Despite the well-documented effects of anger, fear, and anxiety on the ability to reason, many programs continue to ignore the need to engage the safety system of the brain before trying to promote new ways of thinking."[6]

Effective and responsible therapists understand the need for personal and professional growth. Rapid advances in brain science demonstrate the necessity of developing knowledge about the body and physiology—and related skills that often differ from traditional therapy practices. Getting certified as a yoga instructor or making sure you have a solid foundation in yoga is essential to incorporating these skills safely. I hope this chapter and this book help clients and therapists gain an understanding of how important it is to include the body in our work, and get excited about how yoga can be a part of advancing psychotherapy.

As my first yoga teacher stated, "You get one body for this lifetime. Treat it well."

Notes

1 Alexander, F. and French, T.M. (Eds.) (1946) *Psychoanalytic Therapy* (New York: The Ronald Press Company).
2 Siegel, Daniel J. (2007) *The Mindful Brain* (New York: W. W. Norton).
3 Carney, Dana R., Amy Cuddy, and Andy J. Yap. (2015) "Review and summary of research on the embodied effects of expansive (vs. contractive) nonverbal displays." *Psychological Science*, 26(5): 657–63. See: http://faculty.haas.berkeley.edu/dana_carney/pdf_Summary_Expansiveness.pdf (retrieved 5/17/2015).
4 Lazar, S., Kerr, C.E., Wasserman, R.H., *et al.* (2005) "Meditation experience is associated with increased cortical thickness." *Neuroreport* 16(17): 1893–97.
5 Sternberg, E.M., M.D. (2000) *The Balance Within: The Science Connecting Health & Emotions*. (New York: W.H. Freeman & Co.).
6 Van der Kolk, B. (2014) *The Body Keeps the Score* (New York: Viking), p. 86.

12 Yoga for Emotions: Tools for Healing from Eating Disorder Behaviors

Lori Haas

Our bodies are containers and mediums for emotions. When the human brain perceives a threat, the body instinctively goes into fight, flight, or freeze mode. For example, the sympathetic nervous system triggers adrenaline bursts which help the body move quickly—either to battle the threat, or run away from it. These "fight or flight" instincts developed over thousands of generations to promote survival in humans and other species.

Our emotional reactions can be just as powerful when danger is perceived or imagined (you think you see a snake) as when the danger is real (the snake is actually under your foot). Humans often respond to a perceived threat by living in anxiety and fear—even when there is no evidence of imminent danger.

Fortunately, humans have the capacity to allow intense emotions to arise and dissolve naturally, no matter what circumstances trigger them. People grieving after the breakup of a significant relationship might feel a whole range of emotions such as sadness, rejection, fear and loneliness. If they know how to allow, feel, and honor these emotions, even intense feelings will flow through them during the healing process, rather than becoming permanent lodgers.

When we notice a feeling and experience its sensations without a strong attachment to the emotion itself, we are "flowing with emotions." This flow happens by releasing emotional pain through healthy body responses—including tears, connecting with others, retreating, and self-care tools such as journaling, meditation and yoga.

Eating Disorder Behaviors and Emotions

Individuals with eating disorders often respond inappropriately to feelings because the emotions feel too painful, incomprehensible, terrifying, uncontrollable, etc. Instead of flowing with emotions, they often stop the "flow" with eating disorder behaviors that provide a temporary sense of control, relief, comfort, or distraction. Many clients call this "turning down the volume" of their emotions. Turning down "problem" sensations fosters a cycle of symptom behaviors that become entrenched. Furthermore, the expression of positive feelings like love, joy, and peace are turned down too, which affects vibrant relationships and the connection that the authentic self really wants and needs.

Eating disorder behaviors do not allow clear, direct emotional expression and problem solving. The behaviors are a foreign language that the therapist (and, ultimately, the client) must learn to interpret by asking questions such as: "What statement(s) are the behaviors making?" The "translation" helps provide clients with understanding and motivation to learn healthier forms of expressing and experiencing emotions.

How Does Yoga Help?

Eating disorder behaviors can temporarily distract from or release the pressure of intense emotions and bring a sense of relief. They then become habitual patterns, which yoga calls samskaras. Yoga teaches people how to break old patterns and flow with emotions, bringing about relief that improves rather than undermines well-being.

Yoga teaches us how to connect to what we are feeling, thinking, and experiencing in our body *with* compassion and *without* judgment. Yoga develops our skills to deal with triggers and sensations by taking intentional nurturing action, rather than using compulsive or unconscious habits of avoidance, repression, or distraction.

Yoga practice fosters health and healing through:

- A philosophy of no-harm
- Conscious living
- Meditation (focus of healing intention)
- Mantra (conscious, repeated, healing statements)
- Breath that invites and supports what one wants to embrace
- Asana (physical postures/poses)

With these ancient tools, practiced repeatedly on the mat, we strengthen connection with our thoughts, feelings, and actions. In turn, this reinforces a new way of living *off the mat*.

Using Yoga to Shift Mind and Body

Always start by checking in with and discerning the client's needs. Ask clients to notice what they are thinking, feeling and experiencing in their body. Encourage them to link *what* they are feeling with *where* they are feeling it in their body and the pattern of their breath. This cultivates mind-body awareness, reinforcing the knowledge of how feelings are stored in the body.

Yoga reminds us that all our experiences are teachers. Effective yoga practice does not try to eliminate the difficult emotions in a client's affect, posture, and tone of voice. Instead, yoga teaches clients to observe the embodiment of emotions, and learn tools to help the emotions flow and evolve naturally, without judgment. A simple, compassionate statement like, "This is what I am feeling right now" honors the emotion just by observing, feeling, and naming it. This fosters acceptance and brings a sense of safety—opening up the potential for the emotional intensity to soften.

The concept of an internal "observer mind" helps people notice what they are feeling without the need or urgency to react or judge. With practice, yoga develops the "observer mind" to facilitate conscious choices when urges arise. From this place of conscious living, a whole host of positive changes can occur.

Yoga helps us join with our body, rather than making it an unlucky recipient of negativity and disconnection. When in alignment with yoga poses, our postures shift into positions that help the body breathe more effectively—thereby shifting affect, energy, mood and perspective. Breath and posture enhance body awareness, which is a first step toward a positive relationship with the body.

Yoga practice demonstrates how shifts in the ways we use our bodies can create shifts in our emotions and thinking—and vice versa. By learning to change the breath and posture on the mat, the practice retrains the brain and body you take with you everywhere.

Yoga also helps access desirable emotional and relational states by moving the body into a position that illustrates those states. Ask clients to show a body posture that is in alignment with their "happiest and healthiest self." An embodied vision of recovery helps engage all aspects of healing and develops the client's intention and desire for healing—strengthening their healthy self.

Yoga: An Easily Accessible Tool

Yoga breathing and poses enhance (rather than replace) other recovery tools like traditional therapy, nutritional counseling and other treatment modalities. Yoga is an immediate tool for connecting with their body, experience and self when journaling or talking with a psychotherapist might not be an option. Clients can carry yoga's philosophy and practice with them throughout life and through any emotional experience.

Effective yoga practices can be used in a treatment provider's office or studio. For example, breath work, heart openers, or standing poses are simple and easy to do anywhere. Clients could stand in a yoga pose and notice when their body wants to fidget or exit the pose. Suggest that, rather than fleeing the pose, they breathe, stay with it, and become more stable in it, even for a moment. This helps teach the ability to tolerate urges without impulsively acting on them.

Offer suggestions, not prescriptions—helping clients modify poses to suit their needs. For example, standing poses can be done while seated in a chair.

After multiple yoga experiences clients can access their yoga-enhanced muscle memory and sensations visually or literally, when they need to call upon strength, balance, or relaxation. This allows for a healthy and sustainable alternative to eating disorder symptoms.

Specific Poses for Specific States

The following are emotional states common to eating disorders and yoga tools that can facilitate the flow toward healing.

Depressed Energy

The client's posture and breathing are valuable and concrete signals for both therapist and client. A lethargic, depressed person may show up with rounded shoulders, slowed breath and not engaging muscles in their abdominal region. They may describe feeling heavy, pushed down, or weighted in the shoulders. Smiling might be hard since engaging the small facial muscles can seem like a struggle.

Someone with depressed energy may need rest or sleep, because of fatigue. Five minutes without muscle activation in Child's Pose (or another restorative yoga pose) can concretely and immediately provide rest.

Some clients need to *energize* their system. Rejuvenating poses provide lightness to balance the heavy energy of depression. Back bends or inversions are energizing. My clients feel energized when poses balance opening the heart (back bends) and releasing tension (forward folds).

The four-point breath exercise helps depressed energy. In a standing position (mountain pose), inhale from the belly three times so the breath rises to the chest, as the arms extend frontward at shoulder height. Next, move the arms out to the side into a T-position and then overhead. Finally, while vocalizing a big, audible "ha," release the breath while bending forward with the knees slightly bent. Three sets of eight repetitions in a somewhat rapid, but safe flow will energize the body. (Stimulating breath is not indicated for someone in a manic state.)

A gentle Flow style can train the mind to stay present, because the client focuses on connecting each movement with the full length of the breath. Other classic sequences for overall energizing are Sun Salutations A and B. Some clients build toward practicing these flows three to five times a day.

Anxious Energy

Anxiety is the body's reaction to discomfort, pain and fear, whether perceived or real. Because anxiety activates the sympathetic nervous system, the client may experience it as clenching in the stomach and chest, rapid heart rate and/or shallow breathing.

Someone with anxiety may have a rigid posture and stance—physically and emotionally. Tightly rounded shoulders may attempt to protect the heart by closing it off. The person may feel "paralyzed" while the intensity of anxiety is trapped in their body container. People with anxiety may also feel like their "skin is crawling" or they are going to "jump out of their skin," even though they may appear calm to an observer.

Others with anxious energy may appear to be in an adrenaline-fueled, "overdrive" mode of perfectionistic tendencies and anorexia and/or over-exercising behaviors. Stress hormones adrenaline and cortisol surge in response to critical, self-attacking thoughts of the eating disorder self. The resulting anxiety produces an internal trauma environment which weakens the body.[1] "Overdrive" activities may give a false (and temporary) sense of calm, but in the end, anxious energy creates more anxious energy.

With anxious clients, I may start with a gentle Flow style that includes standing poses (such as Warrior A, Warrior B, Reverse Warrior, etc.) to meet the anxious mind where it is in the present moment. The transitional movements from pose to pose release kinetic energy before we slow down the Flow sequence as the mind becomes calmer. We then move onto the floor and use restorative poses to practice the relaxation response.

I always end these sequences in savasana or Corpse Pose to bring stillness. Savasana re-trains the brain and body to experience restoration after movement bringing the yin (calm/nurturing energy) to the yang (stimulating, active energy). Savasana can be extremely challenging for people with anxiety (most eating disorder clients) because they are not used to stillness. If a client struggles to stay still in savasana for more than a minute or two, I don't force it. I also teach breath and mind-focusing skills during savasana to help clients build to longer periods of restoration, as much as 20 minutes a day, with or without other yoga practice.

Restoration is vital on and off the yoga mat. It elicits the parasympathetic nervous system's calming response, which reduces cortisol. This improves sleep quality, increases mental clarity, strengthens the immune system, reduces food cravings, improves appetite, and improves overall health.

A Body Anchor tool helps to ground or "anchor" the healthy experience in the body. For example, Child's pose can effectively calm the nervous system and anchor relaxation into the body and mind. I have clients hold this pose for three to five minutes with the muscles disengaged and the breath flowing freely. On the exhales, I emphasize releasing any tension through the finger tips.

The balancing and calming tool "Bilateral Stimulation Flow" (BLS) also helps to connect logic and emotion centers in the brain. BLS is an important element of Eye Movement Desensitization and Reprocessing, which shows success in healing anxiety and trauma, common issues in eating disorders.[2] Using BLS in yoga, I introduce a Butterfly Hug (arms crossed, giving themselves a gentle embrace) while standing and swaying back and forth from left to right. I invite clients to bring in a mantra ("All is well" or any other healing expression) and then couple it with the breath to ground loving energy into the body. The swaying side to side movement also works well with Seated or Standing Half Moon pose.

A breathing exercise (pranayama) for anxiety is nadi shodhana, or alternate nostril breathing. Start this balancing breath by inhaling through the left nostril while gently closing the right nostril with the thumb. Then, use the ring finger to close the left nostril while the exhale releases out of the right nostril. Repeating the pattern about eight times calms the nervous system. Another, more traditional version, balances the nostril breathing by alternating the inhales and exhales.

Fearful Energy

Fear-based living shows up in our clients' posture and breath. One of my favorite yoga therapy practices is to ask clients to place their body in a position that depicts what it feels like when they are active in their eating disorder behaviors. I call this the ED asana (or Eating Disorders pose). Most folks place their bodies in a closed position, for example, curled up like a ball or in a fetal position.

When I ask them to peek up and see how they are connected with the world, it is quite apparent that they aren't. In this moment, they are consciously embodying their "disconnection" process.

Next, I have the clients move from ED asana into grounding poses. I might have them shift into a forward fold, where they remain curled in a fetal-like position—but with their feet solidly on the ground. I invite them to notice their breath, and how it is slowed because of the body's clenched, frozen and fearful stance.

Next, I have them roll up through the spine into standing position, perhaps with a slight back bend as they lift their arms overhead. From this pose, I ask them again to notice their breath and how they connect with the world. Of course, this open stance may be scary at first, but they now have the direct experience of going from closed/frozen/fearful/disconnected to openness—a position where the breath flows freely. With this simple sequence, the client can feel more connection with the others and the world.

Arching the back expands space in the chest and lung area, opening the heart. The resulting sensation may feel uncomfortable at first, but it makes the energy of love, joy, and compassion more available. One of my favorites is Sphinx pose. The bent back compresses the area around the kidneys—which yoga believes is an organ that holds fear. When the client releases the back bend, blood rushes to nourish the compressed area helping release energy and bring restoration.

To embody empowerment, Warrior B is a strong Body Anchor. The leg muscles are activated, the feet rooted to the ground, and the spine feels lengthened. I add a gesture (abhaya mudra) where the right hand is raised to shoulder height, arm bent and palm facing outward to denote "fearlessness." I also use variations with the palm facing inward, to help clients symbolize the ability to face fear, or the courage to stand up to the eating disorder's critical mirror and start embracing the body.

Anger Energy

Outward expressions of anger are often displayed in a raised voice, clenched jaw or fist, inflated or "puffed" out chest and a wide, fighting stance. Anger energy frequently heats up the body, hence expressions like, "That makes my blood boil!" Anger activates the psoas muscle deep within the abdominal area, so that the hip flexors are prepared to power the legs into fight or flight.

For some people with eating disorders this *outward* expression of anger may manifest in purging and excessive exercise—harmful forms of stimulating energy and physical release.

The *inward* expression of anger can be visible in a frozen smile, rigid stance, or flat affect. Compulsive overeating, food restriction and other eating disorder behaviors can cover up or distract from anger. For example, a client's unspoken message may be that "I am angry at you, but I can get back at you by not eating." Meanwhile, people-pleasing can be a dishonest expression of anger (especially in response to unmet needs) and passive-aggressive behaviors turn suppressed anger into a form of self-punishment, while indirectly signaling others.

Yoga can help clients identify the emotion in their body, accept it, and release it constructively.

One of my "go to" yoga tools is having clients take a big inhale while lifting their arms up over their heads while seated or standing. Then, on the exhale, they flick their wrists several times as they bring the arms back to their sides. The simple movement allows the body to experience a full breath from the belly (eliciting a calming response)—an alternative to the intense, shallow, chest-only breathing which stimulates anger energy. The wrist flicking helps release unwelcome energy, as if flicking away a mosquito. Simple variations can help, too—such as bending the knees on the exhale, and then straightening up on the inhale into a slight arching of the back. I also find it effective to add vocalization of words and phrases such as "let go" on the exhales.

For instance, we use what my clients and I call F-U yoga. When I introduce this concept, clients laugh because they don't usually equate yoga with anger or foul language. F-U yoga involves doing a simple flow sequence (like the Sun Salutations A and B) while yelling words that reflect the intensity of the client's anger energy.

As we begin, I say: "If your anger had a voice, what would it say?" This sets an intention for their voice to express what they really want to say to or about the people and/or situations triggering their anger. Some folks curse, while others just grunt or growl. Usually the anger is released within a few moments—and some clients experience additional relief from the *explicit* permission to be angry.

To embody strength and empowerment I have clients stand in Warrior A pose while pressing their hands, at shoulder height, into a wall or against a partner. People who typically stuff or reject anger often have a tough time with this at first.

Before getting into the pose I ask: "How are you feeling? Where do you feel the anger sensation in your body?" I instruct clients to fully ground the feet, engage the leg muscles, activate the core and tuck the tailbone forward. With the shoulders pulled away from the ears and down the back, they lift and slightly arch the chest area. This alignment lengthens the spine, naturally integrating sensations of strength and being grounded and creating a positive body memory to access in the future.

Next, I have clients push forward into the pose and notice the heat building in the muscles and body. Often, as they push, I have them vocalize or yell what their anger needs to say. After a few cycles, I instruct the client to gently come back to a standing pose and repeat our "go to" tool (inhaling with arms over head and then flicking the wrists back down to the side of the body on the exhale) several times. This process typically takes five to 15 minutes.

At each pause point, it's important to check in with what clients are feeling and where they specifically sense it in the body. They typically will begin to notice anger (and other emotions) flowing from areas of the lower torso all the way up and out of the mouth.

Yoga replaces compulsive habits with the conscious practice of emotional flow. As clients practice the release of anger energy, other, more deeply embedded emotions, such as hurt and sadness, tend to rise up. When this happens, I reinforce the need to use yoga practice *and* talk therapy to work through the healing process.

Shame Energy

Shame is the internal process of feeling and believing a deep rooted sense of unworthiness and inadequacy. As I explain to my clients, shame ("there is something wrong with me") is much harder to address and dissolve than guilt ("I did something wrong").

Many people with eating disorders use symptom behaviors to relieve the pain of shame, e.g., trying to change their external appearance as a path to being "worthy." Often a false self develops that can be described as the Perfectionist, Judge, Critic or ED (eating disorder). Our goal is to help clients release shame and regain the ability to open themselves to worthiness and their authentic self.

We use a "Sacred Space Warrior sequence" to build on concepts for dissolving shame. We begin in the Warrior B pose, with arms out to the side in a "T" position, and then move into Crescent pose, with hands connected out in front of the body at shoulder height. Next, we venture into a Revolved Warrior B pose, back into Crescent pose, lifting the arms overhead with a mini arch in the back. From here, we exhale with a vocalized "ha," as we complete the sequence by returning to Warrior B. And then, we repeat the sequence.

I recommend moving slowly between poses, and holding each pose for a moment or two to help clients embody the experience. As the client's body becomes more stable in poses and more mobile in the transitions, we can go deeper into both poses and movements. For example, I guide participants to hold a pose while attending closely to their breathing and working to lengthen each inhale and exhale. Clients also appreciate adding a clear image or mantra—such as, "I matter" or "I am powerful"—to embrace self-worth and their authentic self.

Shame usually involves thoughts like: "I do not matter" and "I don't have a right to take up space—or even exist." Yoga practice fosters the dissolution of shame by creating space and experiences that embody the person's worth and right to be alive. The space our body occupies is an important concept here.

Have clients visualize their yoga mat as a simple, physical, sacred space symbolizing a healthy, safe boundary around the body. Help clients use this external boundary concept connecting it with the right to take up space. They can engage in activities where they need to express when another person is, or is not, allowed in their space—an embodiment of healthy boundaries.

Embracing the Authentic Self

Through practices of self-compassion and self-acceptance, yoga helps people let go of the false self and develop the skills needed to connect with the authentic self—a self which befriends the body. Yoga builds on our clients' inherent value to develop momentum, motivation and empowerment that are greater than the force of their shame and fear.

One client with a history of significant trauma, anorexia, anxiety and depression presented with a closed off posture and hid behind her hair (a stance of shame). A gentle Flow style yoga met her anxious mind-body with movement and breathing, which allowed her to be present. For instance, we moved from Mountain Pose (to feel grounded standing) to a Standing Forward Fold (to surrender and release) to Chair Pose (feeling strength and opening the heart, while holding her vision of healing in her hands over head), before returning to Mountain Pose. We also used a sequence of restorative yoga poses—and always ended with savasana. With greater body, mind and emotion connection, this client reported feeling more empowered overall, and still uses sequences or distinct poses when needed.

To help embrace one's true self try adding the Lotus mudra to poses. This is a hand gesture made by connecting the thumbs and pinky fingers together while the base of the palms touch and the rest of the fingers open so they look like a lotus flower blossoming. The symbolism is rooted in the way lotus flowers grow toward the sun from dark, murky water, and then unfold into radiant blossoms. Using this gesture during poses while being conscious of its symbolism, embodies the idea that recovery is like moving from darkness (worthlessness) to lightness and enlightenment (worthiness).

Yoga helps people experience their capacity for power and choice, thereby embodying the worthiness already existing within them. Repeated exposure increases the willingness to accept their worthy self and release the shame-filled version.

Overflowing Emotional Energy

Shedding tears and expressing pain while grieving can be healthy ways to allow the natural flow of emotions. Acceptance of the flow actually *honors* the emotions, facilitating their release, and allowing healing energy to arrive.

On the other hand, some people lose (or never develop) the ability to deal effectively with emotions. Their feelings sometimes flood out in a chaotic dysregulated way one moment, only to repress emotions the next. In treatment and therapy sessions, vacillation in behavior and stance can signal overflowing emotions swinging from one extreme to the next. We see some clients, on an unconscious or conscious level, use their emotions to get attention or desired responses from others. People nearby may feel hijacked and drained by this "energy vampire" behavior.

Yoga focuses on "releasing and renewing"—grounding floods of emotional energy within the body container with nourishing breath, posture and mindset. From this foundation, we learn to release stressful energy and emotions which are not serving us well.

An effective yoga tool for overflowing emotional energy is "Taoist Breathing." With feet about three feet apart and toes slightly turned outward, bend the knees as the arms cross near the belly area. On the inhale, straighten the legs, return to standing, lift the arms overhead, and then exhale while crossing the hands behind the neck. Continue the motion by thrusting the arms out into a T position to symbolize "releasing anything that is no longer serving me." Focus on any tension leaving from the finger tips while releasing energy with a big "ha" sound.

Next, bring the hands down crossing near the belly again while bending the knees—but this time, touch the hands together with the thumbs and index fingers connecting like a downward facing triangle. Lift the hands and arms overhead from the navel up through the mid-line of the body with a big inhale to focus on welcoming a vision of new, positive, healing energy. Then return in the same way from the crown of the head down through the mid-line of the body to "ground" with a renewal of positive energy ending at the navel point. Practice this round several times until a feeling of tense energy is "released," new focused and positive energy enters the brain, and the body feels renewed.

"Chair Twist" also clears out old emotional energy. First, the inner organs are compressed. Then, when the twist is released, fresh healthy blood flow goes into the "squeezed" area. Twists also point the body in different directions that encourage a new emotional and symbolic perspective. Begin the Chair Twist while in Chair pose (utkatasana), or, if necessary, while sitting in a chair. Bring the palms together into "prayer" position and move the hands to the heart center. Now, twist the torso so that the left elbow is outside of the right knee. The gaze is backward, so this is a good moment to ask: "what was your old way of viewing things?" Next, ask clients to open up to "a new way of thinking" as they release the twist with a big inhale while lifting the arms overhead as the body settles back into chair pose. This helps ground a new perspective. Repeating the twist to the other knee completes the sequence.

Sometimes I have clients vocalize their new, positive view, and imagine holding it up between their hands. Bringing the hands back to the heart center also helps ground the new vision. This experience embodies the idea of shifting perception (a path to liberation) rather than staying stuck in old ways of feeling and seeing the world and their body.

Tools for Disrupting Eating Disorder Urges

Clients in treatment and early recovery frequently struggle with strong urges that pull them toward their destructive eating disorder cycle. Providers and clients can use any of the tools above to disrupt urges and regain focus on healing and higher consciousness. Encourage clients to experiment with specific poses or sequences to discover what is most effective in specific circumstances.

Hips and shoulders frequently store a lot of tension, tightness, and past emotion. I use poses and sequences that rotate the hips in "release" movements. The discharge of muscular tension through yoga frequently leads to the therapeutic release of feelings—even to the point of cleansing tears that facilitate a beautiful and flowing release of emotional pain. A client recovering from anorexia and bulimia, with anxiety, depression and over-exercising tendencies said: "This yoga unlocks emotions that I have tried to push down for a long time. It seems to happen when we are working on postures that open the hips."

This client credited the yoga process with fostering her ability to tolerate, stay present, and make better choices even when negative thoughts or intense emotions arose. She learned to pay attention to her body, thoughts, and feelings—honoring them and knowing that what she feels will pass.

Inversions also stimulate energy and bring clarity. Anytime the head is below the heart, fresh blood flows to the brain. This can help a person re-evaluate a situation giving them time to respond differently. Common partial inversions like Downward Facing Dog also strengthen and stretch the body.

Love and Joyful Energy

What do you notice when someone is in love or exuding joy? Their face is vibrant and they radiate positive energy. They feel inspired and connected, while experiencing joy and gratitude within their body. In response, other people feel inspired and connected in their company.

I've seen yoga help eating disorder clients visualize emotional and relational states—like love, connection, and joy—which they *want* to experience. Through yoga, I can encourage clients to look at the people, places, things and mindsets that might help them feel sustained brightness and peace. Working with that vision, we can learn ways to focus energy in that direction— instead of toward the people, places, things, and mindsets that deplete and endanger us.

The posture of someone living from a joy-filled place is typically "in alignment." The body feels simultaneously grounded to the earth and lifted through the spine as if connected to the sky. This lengthened posture lets the breath flow freely, and holds the body in a balanced, open hearted stance. The gaze looks straight ahead or slightly upward, demonstrating how the body-mind views life from a place of gratitude and serenity—open to receiving connection and joy.

I invite clients to start embodying this by shifting to the stance (posture and breath) of someone living in connection and joy. Clients' willingness to adopt this stance begins to alter their perception of life, helping them see it through the lens of love and compassion.

I use several yoga tools to cultivate love and joy. First, a "Moving Mantra" starts with asking the client to visualize what love or joy would look like in words, energy, or experience. Next, invite them to experience this visualization in their body, noticing how the breath breathes and how the body feels. Have them narrow the experience of it down to one word. For example, most people say some variation of "peace" or "light."

Next, have clients bring their word into a mantra or affirming statement, e.g. "I am peace." Then introduce a simple yoga movement, such as Warrior A, to embody peace. With the top of the hands over the third eye (located between the brows), have clients say the word "I" (connecting to higher consciousness), followed by "am" as the legs straighten on an inhale, with the arms circling out like a big sunshine. Finally, move back into Warrior A with the hands on top of each other at the heart center (solidifying the mantra into the heart) as they say the last word "peace." Practicing this helps clients feel the energy of the words they are verbalizing.

Turning up the volume of love and joy generates new energy and new ability to embody what we really want to be feeling and how we really want to live. As the spiritual author Marianne Williamson puts it: "A miracle is just a shift in perception from fear to love."[3] The energy of love is more elevated or feels lighter in nature, which can challenge the heaviness of fear or any other obstacles. Another higher vibration energy flows from the practice of gratitude. Bringing gratitude into any situation has the potential to melt away non-serving emotions.

After months of yoga therapy and psychotherapy, a client with anorexia nervosa and intense anxiety described how changes in her posture improved her powers of observation. She described walking around her college campus with a new found way of seeing the world. "It was like all of my senses were so vibrant in taking in my experiences, that I'm seeing beauty in everything I look at." She was embodying and solidifying her capacity to live from a joyful and connected place.

Summary

I believe that:

- Full recovery of an eating disorder is possible.
- Using yoga *along with other healing modalities* helps recovery happen.

Yoga's simple tools of poses, breathing, vocal expression and mindful intention help eating disorder clients learn how to recognize what they are feeling, express it, and then release it. In the end, they feel calmer in the body and perceive greater insight.

I encourage clients to try yoga therapy for 10 sessions and journal about the changes they notice in their bodies and selves. Clients who complete this recommended path tell me they experience a shift in posture and awareness, along with release from old ways of thinking and feeling. They illustrate how direct yoga practice on the mat translates into their lives off the mat and in recovery. They feel more alive, because they are living in—and nurturing—their authentic selves. Transformation happens.

Notes

1 Sarno, J.E. (2007) *The Divided Mind: The Epidemic of Mindbody Disorders* (New York: Harper Perennial).
2 Shapiro, F. (2013) *Getting Past Your Past: Take Control of Your Life with Self-Help Techniques from EMDR Therapy* (Emmaus, PA: Rodale Books).
3 Williamson, M. (1996) *A Return to Love: Reflections on the Principles of a Course in Miracles* (New York: HarperOne).

13 Embody Love: How Yoga Teachers Help Prevent and Treat Eating Disorders and Negative Body Image

Melody Moore

What can today's yoga teachers do about the ways that mainstream yoga classes contribute to, rather than ease, body image despair and eating disorders? How can we avoid the pitfalls that arise when people with eating disorders and/or body image despair join our classes? Can today's yoga teachers be of service by bringing yoga into an eating disorders treatment program? If so, what tools are essential when we work alongside people struggling with these complex illnesses?

Whether in studios, treatment centers, or non-traditional settings, yoga teachers work with people who inflate the value of their external appearance. Whether we realize it or not, yoga teachers also work regularly with people who have disordered eating and/or body image distress.

As yoga instructors, we have the responsibility to understand our impact on these students. We can positively influence self-image and body image for ourselves and those we serve. This means learning how to respond in ways that "do no harm," and knowing how and when to encourage students to get appropriate help and support.

This chapter describes a teaching philosophy called Embody Love Yoga (ELY), an adaptable approach that yoga teachers, yoga studios, therapists and treatment programs can use for people struggling with eating disorders and body image despair.

When touching the lives of people with a severely disconnected sense of mind and body, we must rely on a systematized yoga theory and perspective that gives us knowledge, practice and metaphor for creating balance, flexibility, presence, connection and compassion.

Like yoga itself, the elements of Embody Love Yoga require honesty. They especially demand a fearless assessment of the assumptions underlying our training as yoga teachers—and our own struggles with inflating the value of external appearance, negative body image and/or eating disorders. Our students' healing and hope require that we first engage in transparent, reflective and authentic investigation of our own responses to our own bodies and minds.

From Theory to Application

In 2010, I wrote and offered a seven-week yoga and psychotherapy curriculum for eight adolescent girls with eating disorders. As a clinical psychologist specializing in treating eating disorders, I felt like I'd found a missing link in recovery. Teaching my clients to embody their experiences created a connection between their severed cords of mind, gut and heart—giving us a way to help them reconnect and recover.

After years of not being able to identify her body's hunger and fullness signals, one client responded to a deep breathing exercise (ujayi pranayama) by saying: "I can't believe it; I feel hungry!" Reestablishing connection with belly sensations gave her access to what her belly needed. She wasn't alone. Every one of those eight clients stopped engaging in eating disorder symptoms, no longer views her body negatively, and no longer values herself based on her external appearance. Most practice yoga regularly and two are now registered yoga teachers.

I then worked on additional ways to connect the practices of psychotherapy and yoga, so that more people could use this powerful combination for eating disorders prevention and treatment. I began to train other yoga teachers to apply an approach called Embody Love Yoga (ELY), a practice that:

1 Promotes deep connection to internal experience and opens your body to release emotional tension in a safe, contained way.
2 Introduces you to the gift of intentional breathing, which opens your capacity to sense hunger and fullness.
3 Allows you to be present to and curious about your experience, rather than sitting in judgment of it.
4 Provides safe practice in letting go of expectations, outcomes, and perfectionism.
5 Creates a dialogue for you to sense your own internal critics, which tend to compare your performance to people around you, past experience, and/or external ideals.
6 Allows you to find balance and calm within.
7 Provides you the ability to feel grounded.
8 Helps you use yoga as a tool—on and off the mat—to relieve and release discomfort when you become short of breath, stressed, and/or feel an urge to distract or anesthetize.
9 Invites you to experience your body as connected, whole, and perfect exactly as it is—without the need to change anything.
10 Provides an experience of the surrender of control, not fearing scarcity, not grasping to obtain—but instead allowing the body and mind to release and to rest.

When yoga teachers attend Embody Love Yoga trainings, we begin with a set of welcoming expectations:

- You have chosen to be part of a movement to create safe and sacred space for students and/or clients who choose to practice the art and science of yoga as a way of living in love with themselves and others.
- We will do this by helping students to:

  - Feel their emotions without fear or judgment.
  - Still and calm their minds so that they can observe, witness, and create room for possibility.
  - Develop connections between their physical body, emotional body, mental body and spiritual body.
  - Practice being fully present in each moment.
  - Accept themselves just as they arrive without comparison.
  - Let go of attachment to outcomes, postures, or goals.
  - Experience forgiveness of their bodies, their past and other people.

- Our work will build from the certainty that asana practice is not the end goal, but a tool to finding peace, acceptance and presence.
- We believe that yoga is a state of missing nothing. This belief is fundamental because our students and/or clients often feel as though they are missing many essentials: the perfect body, the capacity to feel their emotions, the ability to be the best and/or a connection to something outside of themselves.
- In teaching yoga, we share the wisdom of connecting mind, body and spirit. We use the practice of asana as a metaphor for the practice of life off the yoga mat.
- We use yoga practice to inform us of the places where we are disconnected or misaligned so that we can bring ourselves into integrity.

Embody Love Yoga welcomes students and clients *as they are* when they arrive. Because every human being yearns to connect and belong, ELY leaders strive for an authentic nature that welcomes and accepts every body and every capacity into our community.

The Culture

ELY believes that yoga teachers must fully participate in subverting the widespread—and mistaken—belief that beauty is something you see, rather than something you are. We directly confront the larger culture in which both teachers and students live—inundated by media, family and peer messages teaching girls and women that we are objects whose worth is defined by external appearance.

As teachers, we can create specific and new conversations that invite girls and women to think for themselves about how they define worth, beauty and purpose. It's a big shift for most students to feel that nothing about them needs to change in order for them to be lovable and valuable. The change requires practice, patience and a teacher who lives this possibility.

Therefore, a central part of our practice is valuing our own contributions and experiencing our personal power to listen, speak, stand up and show up to heal the world. We share this journey's difficulties and joys with our students and/or clients so they will experience (perhaps for the first time) the truth that they are enough in each moment and unique in the world.

The Individual

In one way or another, people with eating disorders have disconnected or severed the cords that unite their body, mind and spirit. People who under-eat or restrict often lose the capacity to recognize and act on their hunger signals. People who binge or over-eat often cannot locate or respond to the body's signals for fullness. By helping the practitioner experience her body as an informant, yoga can attune the needs of the body with behaviors that meet its disparate needs.

Our body tells us about hunger and satiety. It also accumulates our emotions—the physiological sensations stored in our cellular tissues.[1] These two functions are deeply intertwined, but eating disorders disrupt their natural balance as disordered eaters act out their emotions through symptom behaviors.

Allowing the body to release stored-up emotional tension is vital to separating feelings from food. When yoga and psychotherapy help emotions be sensed, felt, tolerated and finally accepted, there is a freedom in the body.

When people are able to feel their emotions and express them appropriately, they can get their needs met in non-destructive ways. Eating disorder symptoms and negative body evaluation can cease to appear to be the best or only solution to life's difficulties. Instead, people can learn to feel comfortable inside of their skin and at peace with thoughts and emotions that arise.

Table 13.1 (on p. 141) outlines specific ways that yoga's healing properties respond to and replace the symptoms and dynamics of eating disorders. It clarifies the reasons that yoga works so well to bring a sufferer's awareness away from self-loathing and into a practice of self-love.

Cueing Classes in Eating Disorders Treatment

Effective treatment teaches clients to identify and pay close attention to the external and internal phenomena that tend to "set off" a chain reaction of symptoms and other self-sabotaging behavior. Treatment providers use knowledge about "triggers" to help clients identify the patterns of their disorder.

Embody Love Yoga pivots the "trigger" concept toward healing by introducing the metaphor of "cueing." Clients new to treatment believe that they are compelled to react to *triggers*, which they perceive as inherently negative. However, *cues* can be seen as neutral, positive, or negative. This terminology shift helps clients grasp the truth that they have agency to *choose* their responses to external and internal phenomena. It also fosters empowerment and agency required to make beneficial choices.

Table 13.1 Transforming Symptoms with Yoga

Quality	Eating Disorder Symptom	Yoga	Mantra
Control	Wish to control, cling to outcome; rigidity, rules, fear of what will happen next.	Surrender of control, letting go.	"I am safe, I am grounded."
Connection	Disconnection of mind from hunger cues. Severed and/or numbed sensations from restriction or mindless eating.	Reconnection through breath and practice of awareness.	"I trust my gut and listen to the wisdom of my body."
Emotions	Wish and/or compulsion to anesthetize, deny, or diffuse through behaviors. Emotions feel uncontainable and overwhelming.	Every emotion is a physical sensation. Yoga can release physiological tension at the cellular level and create containment.	"Feelings are my compass, they teach me where, when, and how to proceed."
Integrity	Dishonesty, incongruity, and conflict among thoughts, words, actions and feelings.	Alignment of head/heart/gut/groin as illustrated by alignment of bones in poses.	"I am truthful with myself and others. I can be trusted."
Balance	Feeling/believing/perceiving that one is not enough or is too much of something, including size/shape/weight.	Practice brings surrender in ways that promote a sense of "enough."	"I am enough."
Mindfulness	Emotionally, psychologically and/or kinetically absent; disassociated.	The intricacies required to approximate certain poses require focus and presence which creates awareness.	"I am here. I am an observer and a witness of myself."
Self-perception	Distorted; overly negative self-evaluation.	Embodied experience of how the body feels and works vs. how it looks.	"My body is a miracle. My body works for me and teaches me."
Acceptance	Comparison of self to others, an ideal, the past, or the future.	Practicing unconditional acceptance of one's pose in the moment.	"I am exactly where and what and who I need to be in this moment."
Boundaries	Enmeshed (cannot distinguish emotional state from others), symbiotic (merges with others), and/or overly rigid (does not trust others)	Knowing when to say "no" and when to ask for support.	"I know how to keep myself safe and choose to ask for help when I need it."
Purpose	Depression, worthlessness and shame; a sense of not having meaning or not mattering to others or to the world.	Connection to sources outside of self, sense of oneness with others and sense of individual capacity.	"I am important. I am valuable. I can create change in myself and in the world."

In ELY classes, teachers invite students to find acceptance and practice self-care. These cues relate directly to key elements of yoga—and recovery. We set up an external atmosphere of safety, acceptance and openness that students can replicate internally on and off the mat. We carefully consider our cues for breath, alignment and lines of energy to help students feel grounded. We consistently remind students to use the practice itself as metaphor and tool for self-inquiry, cueing the exploration of sensations and emotions in the present moment.

Surrender

Most people who struggle with disordered eating are riddled with anxiety and fear of the unknown. Anxiety creates a need to feel in control, predict outcomes and cling to reliable "knowns."

In response, we provide cues for the practice of surrender—the gradual letting go of a specific outcome or result. For example, we bring the student into a half pigeon pose, and then cue her to surrender into the sensation and the stretch. We openly discuss her other options: running away from the discomfort, pressuring yourself to "perfect" the pose, straining and battling your body, etc. This perspective cues the student to understand and embody surrender as essential to progressing in the pose.

We bring students' attention to how they may hold their breath, clench their jaws, or tense other muscles while in a difficult pose. Cueing them to let go of the tension also invites surrender and openness.

Many students with eating disorders resist resting during class—so we explicitly invite them to enter child's pose whenever they are tired, no matter what the rest of the class is doing. This helps them to surrender the outcome of a "perfect" practice or a "perfect" pose. With enough repetition, they can apply this capacity to other areas of life.

Many students are so uncomfortable with letting go of control that they struggle to feel safe and grounded in savasana, or corpse pose. This may seem counterintuitive to people *without* eating disorders who may embrace simply lying down and surrendering all muscular tension, breath control and active thinking. We encouraging students with eating disorders to stay through savasana for at least five minutes because it can profoundly increase their ability to experience themselves as able to surrender their striving to do more, have more, or be more in order to feel safe.

On and off the mat, surrender increases our capacity to release anxiety and strengthen trust in oneself, others, the universe and a higher power or God.

Connection

People with eating disorders damage or sever connections between their minds and bodies. They set up rigid rules about how to feel, when to feel and what feelings are okay or taboo. They even fear feeling their feelings.

This triggers destructive behaviors to numb or distract from emotions—unintentionally storing toxic emotional, psychological and spiritual tension in the body and further disconnecting the mind from the body.

We frequently cue the idea that emotions are physical sensations which build up tension at a cellular level if not surrendered or "let go." We also explore the paradox of how yoga practice *creates* tension in order to release it. For example, when we hold a bound side angle pose for a few breaths, muscular tension builds up before the limbs—and emotions—unwind.

Once unbound, we can learn to feel the emotions, express them, observe them and let them go. The physiological and psychological rebound effect leads from tension and constriction to openness and expansion as we reduce the tendency to avoid, deny, or run from emotions.

Cueing to feel can teach students to use their emotions as their compass—relying on internal experience to navigate their thoughts and behavior, rather than relying on external triggers or "should."

Integrity

Integrity has two primary meanings: the quality of honesty (e.g., being trustworthy) and the state of being whole and undivided (e.g., a building with structural integrity). Both meanings—and the interrelation between them—make integrity a rich metaphor for reconnection and recovery.

During asanas, ELY teachers use body alignment to help students find the "structural" integrity of a pose. When in alignment, the pose feels easy because the body's parts organically integrate in the pose, clearing a path to mind-body connection, integration and integrity. This helps students honestly sense, feel and think in the pose.

From this embodied yoga experience, we explore how integrity works off the mat. When our head, heart, gut and groin—and what they represent—are aligned, life feels easier and less burdensome. When we are out of alignment in asana or in life, we feel physically burdened, strain to keep our posture, quickly lose our balance and even risk injury. ELY teachers emphasize how being out of alignment produces swift physical, emotional, psychological and spiritual consequences.

We teach integrity of the physical poses—and integrity in the ways students treat and speak to themselves and others *off the mat.*

Balance

In yoga, every student sometimes falls, feels off balance, or struggles to stay in a pose. What a beautiful metaphor for recovery, which entails missteps, challenges and moments of relapse.

We illustrate how to find balance by trusting the body's ability to stay focused, mindful and present. This way, students can find a middle path between what feels like too much and what feels like not enough.

In all asana, we find balance by equally extending and contracting; we reach out to the same degree as we are grounding. We have to let go of something (usually tension) in order to open up something else. Often, we root down with whatever body part is on the mat and reach up with whatever body part is extended. The balance comes from relying on our center as the storehouse of our energy. We pull the energy toward us just as much as we push it away.

Mindfulness

People with eating disorders often lack the capacity to observe their own thoughts calmly and compassionately. In order to experience recovery, it is necessary to develop a witness mind, which helps us distance from our thoughts and learn to regulate them. This witness mind also strengthens our understanding of behavior patterns and their consequences.

Yoga has many ways to help people create awareness of how often their minds are disconnected, untamed, or without witness. By consistently cueing clients to notice their thoughts during asana, we teach them to pay deliberate attention to how their mind works and, therefore, how to navigate it. Starting with the alignment of the physical body, we move toward awareness of the physical sensations, and then finally observe emotional activation and intensity.

For example, we wonder aloud with students through open-ended questions like: "Can you notice what might be going on right before your mind took that break from the present moment? Could it have been that something became uncomfortable, and the discomfort led to checking out or drifting off into something safer?"

We emphasize the value of mindfulness even in the moments of distraction. We cue students to approach discomfort as a gift to be fully experienced, inhabited and cherished: the gift of being present to what is and what is available in the moment.

Self-perception

To help shift distorted and harmful perceptions about self, body and inherent worth, we cue eating disorder students to use the rate and depth of their breath to determine the expansion or modification of a pose. This simple invitation can move students from what they think the pose "should" look like to what they are experiencing *inside* their bodies. The perception that a pose should be "perfect" is eventually overwritten by the belief that a "perfect" pose is full of breath and ease, regardless of how "advanced" our execution may be. Asana feels expansive and free when poses are guided by attention to internal experience.

We always recommend working in a space *without* mirrors because they often distract and stimulate over-evaluation and critique. If the only space available has mirrors, we regularly cue students that the yoga experience is not about dissecting or criticizing external images. We invite students to close their eyes in order to navigate through their *internal* perception of and experience in their posture. We also have students adjust their posture, rather than having teachers help "correct" them.

Our goal is building the students' capacity to value who they are and how they feel over what they perceive themselves to look like in a mirror or in other people's eyes.

Acceptance

When people with eating disorders enter a yoga class, they usually have a sense of themselves as unacceptable. They may be afflicted with pervasive and overwhelming feelings that people (including themselves), places and things are not what they ought to be. Paradoxically, the refusal to accept themselves and situations as they are creates greater discomfort, tension and internal conflict.

Yoga is a practice of acceptance—a truth which can be hard for people with eating disorders to tolerate. They often have assumptions about which of their body "parts" don't measure up to the culture's ideal. They may have an "ideal" body or yoga pose in mind. They need guidance into under-standing that there is no ideal person, practice, or pose. Instead, we invite students into experiences where they come to see that how and who they are, right now, is all of the information they need—and is perfectly acceptable.

For example, students often strive to get into a difficult pose variation before they are ready—based on the assumption that anything less (such as a modified variation) is not acceptable. Even when we cue students to accept where they are in a pose and to breathe into the space they find, they may still say to themselves: "I will be acceptable when I can touch my toes, or when I don't have to get into child's pose during an entire class, etc." This thinking pattern is similar to how these students approach body image: "My shape or weight will not be acceptable until I change my ... (fill in the blank)."

We gently remind them that sacrificing alignment in order to achieve a shape means losing the opportunity to experience the pose itself. Instead, when students can accept, in the moment, where they are within the journey of the pose, they can embody the experience as a metaphor for accepting aspects of the self as they are, including physical form.

During sun salutations, we have students inhale the word "I" and exhale the world "Am" as a practice. This consistently reminds students that they are enough—being present is all that is needed. Nothing more is required.

Accepting ourselves does not mean that things cannot change; in fact, accepting where we are helps us to see if and how we can change. To change a pose or a position I have in life I must know where I stand now. We invite students to incorporate this principle into how they view their bodies and, ultimately, into the way they perceive and accept themselves.

Boundaries

We need healthy boundaries for a sense of safety and to guide our choices in life. People with disordered eating often have unbalanced or dangerous boundaries with food, eating, relationships and their bodies. Some don't know what a healthy, self-caring boundary looks or feels like.

To embody healthy boundaries we assure students that they are their own experts. We cue them to "stay on your mat in your own practice, guided by your own experience." We remind students not to compare or compete with what happens on the mats around them: "Ultimately, your balance is not impacted by your neighbor falling over. Nor is your confidence impacted by your neighbor's posture, even if you believe it is more or less 'advanced.'"

Yoga teachers must also attend to our own boundaries by actively attending to how students relate to us. If they attempt to impress or please us, their own practice will suffer. Inquire about any feelings towards you that may come up in class such as:

- Are they angry that you "kept" them too long in an uncomfortable position?
- Do they think you are frustrated, pleased, or disappointed by them?
- Are they "loving" you for your praise, or idealizing you because of your "advanced" practice?

Ask questions *aloud* to encourage students' curiosity and ability to own and share their experience.

Teachers can model healthy boundaries by not taking students' feelings personally. We remind students that they are in control of how long they stay in a pose and how much energy they put towards it. We are not in charge of their experience on the mat, just as no one else is responsible for their decisions or responses off the mat. We cue students to see a direct link between creating a safe physical boundary on their yoga mat and being able to say "No" to unwanted physical or sexual touch off the mat. We also encourage them to recognize all feelings, and take responsibility for the fact that their emotions come from within.

When working with people who have body image or eating dysfunction, teachers must have acute awareness of their position of power over students, because this population frequently has a history of sexual assault, abuse and/or other exploitation. A safe way to allow students space on their mat is to cue, invite and instruct with your words, only rarely using physical assists.

Physical assists and supports may confuse or violate a yoga student's boundary—even if you ask for and receive permission.[2] A student may not feel safe telling you that they feel uncomfortable with the way(s) that you touch them. We work closely with therapists and other treatment providers to monitor and prevent ways we may unwittingly cause harm, even with the best of intentions.

As students learn to set personal boundaries that keep their bodies and minds safe in their yoga practice, they can apply that practice in relationship to eating, their bodies and other people. When students learn to set appropriate emotional boundaries, they are able to enjoy healthy connection that is neither co-dependent and enmeshed, nor isolated and withdrawn.

Purpose

As yoga teachers, we have a role in helping students recognize and believe that they are full of purpose and possibility. Embody Love Yoga posits that everyone has an unrepeatable, incomparable and unique purpose.

We are filled with joy and awe when we witness the transformation of students as they exchange being captive to *what* they are *doing* and how they look for a focus on *who* they are *being* and how they are feeling. As students learn to identify the ways in which they respond to poses, practices, teachers and themselves, they become better equipped to navigate the overwhelming layers of eating disordered illusion and distortion that kept them from seeing clearly that they have purpose and meaning.

Conclusion

The foundation of Embody Love Yoga is the belief that students can learn to:

- Create a sense of internal safety.
- Surrender rigidity and control of outcomes.
- Feel connected to their internal experience, staying with emotions as they arise.
- See that they are missing nothing, and have everything they need within.
- Live in balance and integrity.
- Develop a sense of self-trust.
- Observe their thoughts, feelings and behaviors as a compassionate witness.
- Experience their body as acceptable and sacred.
- Create and hold healthy boundaries for themselves.
- Recognize and live their purpose.

People with eating disorders need a safe container during yoga class because their lives are fraught with distress over their bodies. As teachers, our own capacity to create a safe container will stem from our feeling of safety and acceptance regarding our own bodies.

All students, especially those with eating disorders, hunger for authenticity, consciousness, and integrity. As a teacher, your own capacity to embody love, compassion and truth will be apparent to your students. They will feel and receive the ways you speak, hold yourself, and treat others. Your commitment to living your yoga will have a profound impact on your students' experience of yoga.

We are not responsible for healing our students, because yoga itself works to heal. We are responsible for offering the gift of pointing the way.

Set intentions before class; invoke prayer; open to rebirth and renewal in your closing savasana; be guided by your own wisdom; trust your own experience in leading students through poses that serve as symbols and reflections of a way of living that is connected, integrated and whole.

We help students to experience their practice as embodied prayer and their body as a sacred temple, deserving of consideration and kindness. Working together, we can help open the door to true recovery from disconnection and disease—and allow sufferers to become present to the gift of life itself in full recovery.

This chapter was adapted from *Embody Love Yoga Teachers Manual*, © Melody Moore, Ph.D., RYT and used with permission. Look for more in Dr. Moore's upcoming book.

Notes

1 See Chapter 12.
2 See Chapter 4.

14 NOURISH Yoga Workshops for Recovery

Robyn Hussa Farrell

As an Experienced Registered Yoga teacher, I've led yoga workshops for people with addictions and/or eating disorders for nearly a decade—always working in partnership with trained therapists. Eating disorders are complex, paradoxical and counter-intuitive. This means that yoga teachers cannot take an "ordinary" yoga class and transfer it, unaltered, into eating disorders treatment programs.

In order to serve effectively, yoga teachers must understand the ways in which "mainstream" yoga classes can reinforce eating disorder attitudes and behaviors. I developed the NOURISH Yoga Workshops for Recovery in order to offer yoga while avoiding common pitfalls and keeping the focus on healing.[1] This work does not, in any way, replace treatment. It is specifically designed for people who are in a stage of active recovery from eating disorders or addiction.

The Framework

NOURISH Yoga Workshops can be adapted to a variety of locations and circumstances. You only need 90 minutes and a yoga mat for each participant. The general format includes these elements:

- Free-writing
- Pranayama (breathing) technique
- Gentle asana exercises
- "Workbook" activities such as writing, drawing, arts, partner activities, etc.
- Physical asana (often moderate, but occasionally vigorous)
- Journal writing
- Re-centering with a breathing exercise leading into a short meditation
- Processing

We integrate printed handouts during the yoga practice. The participants read, do work, write, and think while practicing yoga on a mat. There is an intentional and direct purpose for this.

As often as possible, the workshop sessions end with at least 10 minutes of processing with a licensed psychotherapist, so clients can discuss how they will employ self-care in the days ahead.

Engaging in yoga, mindfulness, and meditation exercises guides people inward and helps them listen to their feelings. This can be emotionally flooding for someone suffering from an eating disorder. Yoga teachers are not trained to respond to and contain these complex reactions, so we always have a licensed psychotherapist, trained in eating disorders, on hand to assist. Nevertheless, it is crucial for yoga teachers to understand the co-morbidities associated with eating disorders. Understanding the prevalence of depression, anxiety disorder, trauma history, and more will enable the yoga professional to assist the client in finding greater freedom.

The Environment

Consider practicing in a "neutralized" space, without mirrors or other elements conveying the feel of a dance or workout studio. Clients and loved ones often say that walking into many yoga studios is exceedingly difficult because it re-ignites a competitive focus on external beauty, rather than helping the person remain internal in their validation. The most helpful spaces are areas that evoke the feeling of a calm living room. Most participants prefer to practice in a darkened room with dim candle-like lighting.

Participants should wear comfortable clothes—not necessarily "yoga" attire. I encourage clients to wear whatever they want. In fact, we talk about how freeing it is to wear "PJs" to yoga. They learn that they can come to a yoga class without having to look perfect or yoga-fabulous. This concept is a huge part of their journey, and should be discussed readily. The goal is to teach comfort, self-care, and self-acceptance.

Yoga teachers should make sure that participants who are currently in treatment for addictions or eating disorders provide clearance from their medical treatment team prior to participating in yoga or meditation practices. These clients could be seriously at risk for cardiovascular or other medical complications.

Each participant must bring a journal and writing implement to each class or workshop.

Rather than only engaging in physical yoga asana practices, I encourage instructors to create relaxed, Eight-Limbs-based practices, which enhance mindfulness and other healthy coping skills. This is sometimes challenging for eating disorder clients drawn to a more vigorous (and calorie-consuming) workout. Our challenge is to introduce them gently to slowing down, sitting still, and existing in their own bodies without escaping to rigorous activity, talking, or acting out.

Below, you'll find the framework for two workshops, including a "script" for the teacher to follow and/or work from. This is meant to give the instructor ideas to incorporate into the practice and tools for setting a peaceful and serene environment. These instructor "scripts" are indented.

Example 1: Yamas: Five Crucial Poses and Affirmations for Recovery

This work helps clients learn to think about yoga as something other than a form of exercise. By giving a purpose and affirmation to a physical yoga pose, we help those in recovery to think on more than one level at a time.

1 Opening

Begin the class with everyone seated easily on their mats. Distribute the "8 Limbs of Yoga" handout (available at www.YogaAndEatingDisorders.com).

> Exploring the 8 Limbs of Yoga helps us gain a new perspective on so much of our life. The first limb is the Yamas: observances that help us to live with greater integrity and focus. Yamas are not rules, per se, but opportunities to expand our life into one filled with greater clarity and a deeper consciousness. Yamas help us develop the more profound qualities of our humanity and provide us with self-discipline that allows us to head toward the fulfillment of our life purpose or dharma.[2]
>
> The five Yamas are:
>
> Ahimsa: Kindness or Nonviolence
> Satya: Truthfulness
> Asteya: Abundance or Nonstealing
> Brahmacharya: Non Excess or Moderation or
> Aparigraha: Self-reliance or Non-attachment
>
> For each Yama, we will explore a physical pose and work with an affirmation while in that pose.
>
> The affirmations I use during this workshop are simply suggestions— please re-write or choose others if these do not work for you. As with all recovery yoga, always consult with your care provider or therapist to discuss any thoughts or reactions to this work. Please also keep a journal while you practice.

2 Pranayama Practice: Three-part Breath

Invite the participants to sit on the mat with their legs crossed.

> Relax for a moment or two and slow your breath down. Please make sure your chin is down slightly, back of your neck open. Relax your eye gaze. Relax your jaw, your muscles in your face. Focus only on breathing through your nose and travel the breath all the way down to

your lower back. Then, allow the air to float back up in slow motion as it travels back out of the nose. Imagine the air is like a stream that continues past this room, outside of the building and beyond.

(Repeat this for 3–5 breaths)

In yoga, the art of breathing is called "prah-na-yama" which means "life-force-lengthening." Breathing itself is an act of yoga—uniting our bodies, minds and spirits. Even as we actively practice something as simple as breathing, we are practicing mindfulness. We are uniting; connecting to the breath within the breath—or spirit. This can be whatever the word means to you. For the next moment, then, let's simply contemplate the concept of the breath—or life force—within us.

(Continue for 3–5 breaths)

3 Centering Meditation

From this place of stillness, please close your eyes and bring to your mind a spot on your forehead, just between your eyes. As you focus on your breath, imagine that spot turning a beautiful blue color. Slowly draw in a breath, imagining the blue spot growing to the size of a quarter. Continue focusing on the spot and imagine that it grows with intensity and rich-ness—your favorite shade of blue. Now imagine that color blue extend-ing throughout your body. Imagine a blue sphere enveloping you from the top of your head to the tips of your toes. Take this moment of silence to send a healing thought to your body, your mind and your breath. With gratitude and loving kindness, send the blue healing energy to every cell in your body. When you are ready, open your eyes slowly.

(Please pause for 3–5 breaths)

4 Asana

We move now into practicing gentle asanas as a way to explore the five Yamas. By embodying a physical action symbolically related to a Yama, the student can learn the Yama somatically. This reinforces the use of each pose as a reminder to employ each principle during future practices.

a. Ahimsa: Kindness or Nonviolence—Child's Pose[3]

At root, ahimsa means maintaining compassion towards yourself and others. It means being kind and treating all things with care. One of the main purposes of yoga is to cultivate feeling and awareness in the body. How do we practice non-violence? Towards ourselves when we treat ourselves kindly. How might we treat ourselves kindly? Perhaps we can start by practicing a yoga posture in a way that teaches us loving kindness. I truly believe that if we can practice it on the yoga mat, we can practice it in real life.

Bring the participants into Child's Pose on the mat. Once everyone is settled, invite them to consider the following affirmation:

"I am kind and loving to myself and others."

b. Satya: Truthfulness—Downward Facing Dog

The second Yama is Satya, which means truthfulness. How do you live truthfulness in your life? Practicing Satya means being truthful in our feelings, thoughts, words, and deeds. It means being honest with ourselves and with others.

Bring the participants into Downward Facing Dog. Once everyone is settled, invite them to consider the following affirmation:

"I am learning to recognize and heed the voice of truth in my inner self."

c. Asteya: Abundance or Non-stealing—Warrior II

The next Yama is Asteya, which translates as non-stealing or abundance. Asteya addresses the fear-filled belief that we cannot create or will not get what we need. We steal because we misperceive the universe as lacking abundance; we think that there is not enough for everyone and that we will not receive in proportion to our giving. Asteya helps us recognize that abundance surrounds us and should be embraced with gratitude in all areas of our life.

Bring the participants into Warrior II. Once everyone is settled, invite them to consider the following affirmation:

"I gratefully accept the abundance of health, love and success that surrounds me each day."

d. Brahmacharya: Non-excess or Moderation—Bound-Angle Pose

The fourth Yama is Brahmacharya, which means moderation in all things. The root of the word is "Brahma," which refers to creation. We practice Brahmacharya when we consciously choose to use our life force to express our dharma, rather than to frivolously dissipate it in an endless pursuit of fleeting pleasures. Brahmacharya reminds us that our life force is both limited and precious. This Yama teaches us to use our energy wisely so we can live a fulfilling and meaningful life.

Bring the participants into Bound-Angle Pose. Once everyone is settled, invite them to consider the following affirmation:

"I can and do set limits and boundaries."

e. Aparagraha: Self-reliance or Non-attachment—Savasana or Corpse Pose

The last of the Yamas is Aparagraha which translates as non-posses-siveness, non-attachment, or self-reliance. Rather than looking to find who we are, we often look toward others and strive to emulate them. In essence, Aparagraha helps us discover our own selves so that we no longer feel the need to covet what someone else has, or be what some-one else is. Everything that we need exists within us.

Bring the participants into Corpse Pose. Once everyone is settled, invite them to consider the following affirmation:

"I take full responsibility for all that I am. I am honored to rely on myself, rather than others."

5 *Processing*

At the end of the practice, ask the participants to share their experience and discuss their plan for self-care for the rest of the day and week.

Example 2: What I Want: A Meditation to Enhance Mindfulness

This work is a simple illustration of the peace and centering that yoga and mindfulness can bring to any human being.

This workshop revolves around a "What Do I Want" exercise. The goal is to illustrate the differences we feel inside when we first sit down to ask "What do I want?" early in the class compared to asking the same question toward the end of class, when there is greater relaxation. Are there differences in what a participant wants or desires when they are in a more relaxed state of mind?

Bring yourself and your students into a peaceful, serene state. Perhaps play some tranquil music that facilitates the relaxation process. If possible, dim the lights and/or light a few candles. Speak in a tone that is calming, grounding and peaceful to enhance the client's ability to go "internal."

The goal of this exercise is to teach individuals how their ambitions, desires and needs change as they become more relaxed and centered. Students will need a private yoga journal, a pen and a comfortable place to sit, such as a yoga mat or cushion.

1 Centering

Invite participants to sit on their mats in an easy position ("cross-legged" or "Indian" style). Make sure their yoga journal and pen are within reach.

> Please close your eyes and focus on your breath momentarily. Embrace the potential to have a genuine experience today, in this moment.
> Throughout the course of this yoga practice external thoughts will enter your mind. Please know that these thoughts are natural. Simply acknowledge that these thoughts exist and ask them to leave you in peace as you work on your yoga for the next 15 or 20 minutes.

2 Free Writing

After 15–20 minutes of meditation, invite the participants to "re-enter" the room and take in several relaxed breaths. Next, ask them to open their eyes and immediately begin to free write, emphasizing the myriad benefits of expressive writing.[4]

> For 10 minutes, please free write, without stopping, into your yoga journal about the question or phrase "What do I want?" Allow your mind to run free as you write nonstop and keep your focus on answering the mantra:
> "What do I want?"

3 Re-centering.

Once the free writing exercise is finished, ask participants to set their journals aside and return to an easy seated position with palms together at the heart center.

> Feel your heart beat on the other side of your thumbs or in your fingertips.
> As you relax in this easy seated position, please consider the following quotation from Jon Kabat Zinn's *Wherever You Go, There You Are*:
> "Everything we are in contact with connects us to the whole world in each moment. Things and other people, places and circumstances are only here temporarily. Now is everything.
> It is only by being fully in this moment that any future moment might be one of greater understanding, clarity, and kindness, one less dominated by fear or hurt and more by dignity and acceptance. Only what happens now happens later."[5]
> The way we connect to "now" is through our breath.

4 Pranayama: Samavritti, or Equal-Part-Breath

> We will now practice mindful samavritti ("sa-ma-VREE-tee") breathing or "equal part breath." Samavritti means matching the time or space

it takes to breathe in with the amount of time or space it takes to breathe out.

Begin by simply noticing where your breath is right now in this moment. As you focus on your breathing, be conscious of the amount of time or space it takes to inhale. Then, make this "equal" to the amount of time or space it takes to exhale. You can do this by counting to 4 or 5 or just by feeling how much time or space it takes to breathe in and breathe out. As you work on your samavritti, notice the moment that exists before you breathe in and the moment that exists before you breathe out.

Some say that this is the greatest place of peace that exists in our bodies—the moment before you inhale and the moment before you exhale. Without holding or stopping your breathing, simply notice that this place exists inside of you.

5 *Free Writing for Two Minutes.*

Please now return to your yoga journal (change positions, if your legs are uncomfortable) and journal for two continuous minutes about the idea of "balance" in your life. Where do you find you are "in balance" in your life? Where are you a little out of balance?

6 *Re-centering*

When finished, please set your yoga journal to the side and sit in an easy seated position with your palms face down on your knees to symbolize calm and peaceful energy. We'll take a moment to re-center in our bodies after focusing on our brains to write. Imagine drawing one molecule of oxygen in through your nose and imagine it traveling all the way down to the base of your spine. Allow that oxygen molecule to float back out of your nose as it floats back up past your ribs, past your collar bone and beyond.

7 *Interconnectedness Meditation*

Focus on an image of interconnectedness—the idea that you are an important part of the entire universe. That your being on this planet is no accident. You are here and you deserve to live a life of peace, of happiness, of wholeness. You deserve to feel at home wherever you go. Now please journal one last time about what you want in your life. Set an intention for yourself from this place of internal groundedness and centeredness and please write about it in your journal for the next five minutes.[6]

8 *Processing*

Allow each participant to review and name any feelings that they may be experiencing. You might want to use a visual guide or chart of various feelings in the center of the room to facilitate the discussion. With the guidance of a professional psychotherapist, allow the participants to share their experience and discuss their plan for self-care for the rest of the day and week.

Conclusion

These sessions are effective because they offer practical techniques which clients can apply in real life to reduce anxiety in moment-to-moment experiences. NOURISH Yoga's multiple yoga practices integrate smoothly with the work of therapists, dietitians, physicians, and other professionals trained in the treatment of eating disorders.

Our website of mental health resources[7] provides online trainings on eating disorders awareness and prevention informed by internationally acclaimed researchers who serve as our tribe of medical advisors in prevention and resilience. You can also learn more about eating disorder recovery yoga trainings on the site.

This chapter contains excerpts from *Healthy Selfitude: A Practical Approach to Self-Acceptance Using Performing Arts and Yoga Techniques* and from *Mindfulness & Meditation Techniques for Recovery*, © 2008–2013, whitelephant enterprises. All rights reserved. Reprinted with permission.

Notes

1 For this chapter and NOURISH Yoga practices, I am grateful for the inspiration provided by my mentors Margaret Riddleberger, Laura Lees, Ph.D., CEDS and Debra Hennesy.
2 See Chapter 2 for a full discussion of Yamas and Niyamas.
3 Elements from this section were inspired by Palkhivala, A. (2007) "Teaching the Yamas in Asana Class" posted 8/28/2007 on http://www.yogajournal.com/for_tea chers/984 (retrieved 5/21/15).
4 Gortner, E.M., Rude, S.S. & Pennebaker, J.W. (2006) "Benefits of expressive writing in lowering rumination and depressive symptoms." *Behavioral Therapy* 37(3): 292–303.
5 Kabat-Zinn, J. (1994) *Wherever You Go, There You Are: Mindfulness Meditation in Everyday Life* (New York: Hyperion Books).
6 Inspired by Schiffman, Eric, "Remember to Remember" on *Freedom Yoga: The Art of Living*. http://freedomstyleyoga.com/articles/book-chapters-from-movingin to-stillness/remember-to-remember/ (retrieved 5/21/2015).
7 www.bresilient.co.

15 Three Approaches: Client Perspectives on Strong, Restorative, and Partner Yoga Classes

Elisa Mott

"I am grateful for my nourished soul."

These words were written by my client, Jane, after nearly two years of individualized, one-on-one yoga sessions. When Jane first came to me, her eating disorder was starving her soul. The voice in Jane's head, which she called "Ed," guaranteed the gifts of approval, popularity, and comfort—but only if she purged, over-exercised, and constantly competed against and compared herself to others. Instead of acceptance, "Ed" left her with unquenchable needs and a famished soul.

A growing body of research (including some described elsewhere in this book) shows the positive effects of yoga in addressing body image issues and eating disorder symptoms. However, we seldom read or hear the voice of clients explaining what works about yoga.

I've gathered these voices as a nationally certified counselor, wellness educator and yoga instructor privileged to work with women and men of all ages who struggle with body image, weight, and disordered eating. I've worked with them in an intensive outpatient program and a private, studio setting. No matter the symptoms or level of care, all experienced a deep, incomprehensible emptiness and insatiable hunger in their hearts and souls.

This chapter draws on client evaluations, quotes, stories, and case examples to articulate how these women and men integrated three specific types of yoga classes into their recovery path: Strong, Restorative, and Partner. I have used pseudonyms and eliminated any identifying information about the individuals who describe how yoga deepened their relationship with their mind, body and spirit.

Strong pose classes use asanas which require physical and emotional strength. These poses also provide eating disorder clients with a needed vulnerability to be seen from head to toe.

Restorative yoga classes require more stillness and quietness of mind and body—and therefore allow most clients to feel calmer and more relaxed. The client's body may feel less exposed in restorative practice than in the strong pose practice. However, the active client may find it challenging to remain grounded in a still body.

Partner yoga classes, involve two or more people working together to create the pose. This style of practice assists clients in increased communication, teamwork and proprioception (our sense of the relative position of our body parts and how we perceive the effort we use to maneuver those parts).

Strong Pose Classes

A competitive swimmer and ballerina with anorexia, Susan pushed herself to her edge in every yoga class. She did sit-ups when she thought no one was looking, and held a pose long after the group had come out of it. Her eating disorder demanded ongoing physical challenge to expend calories. For example, she'd say: "I am used to working a lot harder than this. This exercise seems sort of pointless."

Like many clients who struggle with anorexia, Susan was a perfectionist. She wanted to sharpen the shape of each pose, even if that meant straining, holding, and gripping. Having lost much of her muscle strength to her eating disorder, she fought to appear stronger than she really was. I remember one class when, short of breath, Susan trembled to hold an advanced variation of parsvakonasa (a side angle pose) longer than the rest of the group. She looked to me and gasped: "Am I doing this right?"

I invited Susan to a different challenge. "Let's try to imagine what it might be like to practice yoga with only 70 percent of the effort you're giving now. Start to ask yourself where you can pull back and settle into the pose, rather than pushing forward to force the pose."

My mission was to show Susan how classic yoga methods and philosophy emphasize the practice of finding a steady, easeful pose—what yoga philosopher Patanjali called "Sthira Sukham Asanam." Sthira means steady, stable and motionless; sukham means comfortable and filled with ease; asanam means meditation posture. This approach may sound simple, but it isn't easy. While embodying a pose, many yoga practitioners (even those without an eating disorder) struggle to strike a balance between strength, vulnerability and relaxation.

The compulsivity found in people with eating disorders around issues of food and exercise makes it quite difficult to practice mindfulness and ease at *any* moment in time—much less while remaining strong and firm in a yoga pose. My clients are "all or nothing"; either completely relaxed or giving 110 percent to a pose or sequence. Years of symptom use cloud their ability to believe that they can bridge the gap between a meditative practice and a strong practice.

Clients often demonstrate the struggle with comments such as:

- *"I don't find any value in poses like final relaxation (savasana). I'm just lying around. I mean, I can do that at home."*
- *"It's really hard to ease into the poses without giving it my all. If I don't grit my way through it, I feel like I'm failing and like I might even fall out of the pose."*

- *"My eating disorder doesn't believe that yoga is enough for me. It says I'm not good enough, strong enough, thin enough and if I do yoga, I better do it right and burn as many calories as possible!"*

People with eating disorders frequently fear experiences which combine strength and vulnerability. When teaching Warrior II to a group of clients at an intensive outpatient program, I explained that this pose allows you to feel potent and open, resilient and seen.

It's hard for many clients to imagine having any of these sensations, much less all of them at once. As my client LaToya put it, "Being strong means that you're invisible, you aren't bothering or needing anyone. When people pay attention to me, when they finally 'see me,' it's usually because I'm needy, weak and vulnerable."

I encouraged LaToya to imagine great leaders like Martin Luther King, Jr. and Mother Teresa, figures who embodied courage and sensitivity, individuals who touched lives and were touched in return. Yoga teachers and treatment providers need to recognize how challenging it is for eating disorder clients to be and feel seen. Helping them experience strength and vulnerability concurrently in their bodies can be extremely helpful, since their recovery requires that they reclaim their power and become open to developing meaningful relationships.

Strategies like "Let's try this pose at 70 percent or 50 percent" work well in these situations, since our goal is not to push clients to "perfect" poses. Instead, we aim to help clients experience embodiment through poses, breathing, and sequences. That's why instructors need language to explain the difference between exercise and a yoga practice, and then *invite discussion* around the distinction.

After a while, Susan began to understand the concept of 70 percent. She started to practice with the group, rather than jumping ahead to a different pose or taking on a more challenging variation. She slowly embodied santosha, contentment, by holding the pose "within her edge," a stance where she could breathe easy, rest mentally, and open up spiritually. One day, she shared: "Somehow in tandem with others' breath I don't feel selfish. I feel open to possibility instead of trying to force myself to be successful. It gives me permission to just be." In fact, she backed off even more than 70 percent in her Warrior poses and began to embody the essence of Sthira Sukham Asanam.

Clients often admit that standing poses trigger their desire to exercise excessively. Some are surprised or confused when we do standing poses:

- *Isn't this exercise? My doctor and treatment team say I'm not allowed to exercise.*
- *If I'm allowed to do yoga, why can't I also run and go to the gym?*
- *Can I ask how many calories this is going to burn?*

Instructors can leverage these responses to deepen the exploration—and embodiment—of the profound differences between nurturing yoga and abusive over-exercise. In fact, I encourage clients to describe the differences in their own experience. Here are the kinds of things they say:

- *Yoga helps me check in to how my mind and body are feeling and how they are connected—something I've never been able to do before in any other exercise class.*
- *This is pretty much the only time I get to be a little easier on myself.*
- *Closing my eyes helps me a lot to focus, and keeps me from body checking or comparing like I do at the gym.*

Some clients do not have the stamina to maintain strong standing poses for very long. Yoga group leaders must be sure that clients are medically cleared for a standing practice. It is often best for new or fairly weak clients to remain seated at first while doing poses; this can provide a better understanding of the client's experience in her body. During the class, check in for any dizziness or lightheadedness.

However, for most medically cleared clients, standing in the poses is more an emotional challenge than a physical hardship. Why?

Standing poses bring about a sense of vulnerability and concerns about "being seen." Many eating disorder clients believe that the body must not and cannot be seen in full view unless it is perfect and unflawed—an unattainable state. When practicing yoga on the floor, the client can easily hide her body, shrink and cover up. During a standing pose, the whole body is visible, expansive, and noticeable.

Eating disorder clients also may avoid stronger standing poses (and holding those poses) because they are emotionally fatigued, lethargic, or depressed. Once any medical problems are ruled out, the teacher and client can begin an inquiry into why these particular poses are so challenging.

While practicing strength-building yoga poses, Susan heard thoughts such as: "Go deeper, go harder, feel the burn." Ironically, the Sanskrit verb "tap" (which means "to burn") is the root for the yoga Niyama (observance) known as *Tapas*, which means "heat" or "glow."

The mind of someone with an eating disorder is often rigid and overwhelmed with tasks. In contrast, Tapas is achieved by deepening our discipline of stillness and internal focus, in order to quiet the overly active, busy, worrying "monkey-mind." We do not approach Tapas by measuring how low we go in Warrior I or how long we stay balanced in Warrior III. The glow of Tapas comes via the steadiness, consistency and subtleties of our yoga practice. Susan's transformation began when she started to experience the deep, inner fire burning within the chamber of her heart, while also embracing the pose's inner beauty and the stillness of her body and mind.

Strong poses provide another opportunity to light the fire within by using vocalized sounds and words. How does this help the client? The journey to recovery demands that the person find their own unique voice with its own exceptional message and truth. Vocalization during poses can help clients embody their voice, feeling it as a physical sensation.

Our clients are quite familiar with the voice of ED in their head speaking so loud that it drowns out, or even silences, the person's own true voice. The eating disorder self resists efforts to find the authentic self. As my client Madison put it: "If I can begin to turn down the volume of ED and turn up the volume of my own healthy voice, recovery becomes a possibility."

By age 18, Becky had been in and out of treatment multiple times. During our first yoga class together, she cried the entire time. I invited her to stay in class, saying: "As you are able to focus on or be conscious of your breath, you are practicing yoga." For three weeks, Becky remained visibly uncomfortable in her body. She sat on the floor, arms wrapped tightly around her knees, as if in a cocoon. Eventually, she did poses, but tried to appear small and compact, as invisible as possible. She rolled her eyes at my requests or instructions and she could hardly speak without sobbing, so she did not say much at all.

Like Becky, many clients with eating disorders have difficulty expressing themselves without shutting down, numbing out, or crying. Perhaps that is why so many recovered people say: "Finding my voice was imperative to my recovery."

Instructors can be the client's voice by suggesting vocal affirmations. While clients move through poses, I ask them to repeat (silently or aloud) statements such as:

- "*I am strong*" in Warrior pose
- "*I am confident*" in Mountain pose
- "*I am lovable*" in Fish pose

The simple combination of movement and vocalization lets clients "try on" a voice that echoes a new identity of healing and recovery. The instructor states affirmations for the client to hear and repeat. The ensuing sensation invites the client to inquire how she would feel if she were to embody the words (and voice) herself.

I also use the words and metaphors of yoga itself to build internal bonds. When clients are both open and willing, I use *warrior* poses to connect clients to their inner *warrior*. I remind clients how many kinds of warriors there are: warriors of love, of strength and of courage. I ask: "What are you the warrior of today?" When clients are unsure or do not believe they are the warrior of anything, I often prompt them with questions like, "What do you need to overcome today or make peace with today?" I explain that being a warrior incites courage and accomplishment, not aggression or fear.

The resulting exchanges are far more light and fun than you may expect. Adolescents often declare: "I am the warrior of homework!" Working moms triumphantly proclaim: "I am the warrior of traffic." Clients in a treatment program proclaim "I am the warrior of my meal plan!"

As Becky continued to practice and come to class, she cried less and eventually found poses she could hold steadily for longer periods of time. "I'm still uncomfortable and don't really like being in and feeling my body," she said, "but I am able to focus on my breath." She also learned to stay engaged during meditations. During one particularly difficult day, while standing strong in her warrior pose, Becky declared to the class: "I am the warrior of my recovery!"

Another avenue to uncover one's voice, passion and inner fire is to generate unadorned noises. I invite clients to use dragon breath, loud exhalations, grunts, and shouts while in their poses. These simple sounds can ignite Tapas, while simultaneously encouraging one's inner warrior to shine. When we allow sound to release from the body, we also allow energy and air to flow through the body, balancing the chakra associated with fire, courage, and willpower. If this energy is out of balance, we become stubborn, rigid, and closed-off. With balance restored, we find strength in vulnerability and courage in openness.

Susan began to feel this shift, and described it this way: "I want the earth to hold me, rather than hold myself up on the earth." Those words expressed her growing openness to the people and the world around her—as well as a vigorous energy of hope she needs to fuel her journey to recovery.

Restorative Pose Classes

Throughout her life, Sandy endured many traumatic experiences and hated the feeling of being in her body. She struggled with gender identity and dissociative identity disorder. Like Susan, Sandy was accustomed to overworking and over-exercising her body. Nevertheless, her use of extremely gentle, quiet, and meditative restorative yoga steadily had an impact. Gradually, Sandy began to let go of her constant struggle with her body. She began to trust her body in poses and allowed herself to be supported and nurtured in them.

Restorative yoga requires very little physical strength and any size person can do it. Clients are drawn to the inherent safety of prone poses like bala-sana (child's pose), where the person brings their hips to their heels and their forehead to the floor. This creates a boundary around the body, almost as if it is completely protected. I often use guided imagery during restorative yoga. For instance, in balasana, I ask clients to "picture yourself as a small child," and repeat in their mind the affirmation: "I am safe." This feeling of being safely covered up or hidden allows many clients to stay in the pose longer than they might if they felt exposed or vulnerable.

After the client feels comfortable with the instructor and the group, I integrate supine poses, lying on the back. Because these poses leave the stomach exposed, they can be a greater challenge than the "safer" belly-down, prone poses. I increase the feeling of security by encouraging clients to put their legs up on a chair, or by covering the client with a blanket. Many clients enjoy having their legs up on a chair to relieve back tension, while also letting the chair "hold" and support the body.

While Sandy enjoyed the restorative practice, she had days when she struggled with being in her body. She found that seated meditation helped ease the anxiety and discomfort she attached to living in her body. I was surprised by her openness and willingness to engage in meditation; while fidgety at first, she would eventually settle in. Honest about her distractions, she often got frustrated with her "ability" to meditate. She needed constant reinforcement and reminders that meditation is just about noticing; it is not doing mediation "right." After weeks of practicing restorative yoga and meditation, she reported: "During the moments when there is no judgment of myself or my body, there is an absence of nervousness. I feel free in those moments, free of my eating disorder voice, which is the best feeling."

After six months of a consistent restorative yoga practice, another client, Jane, felt transformed:

> *The veil of lies that clouded my vision has been lifted. Without even realizing it, this veil of deception held me back from loving myself and truly engaging with others. The lies I told myself were self-loathing, mean, and competitive. Yoga made it possible for me to slowly awaken, so that instead of constantly comparing and fighting myself, I could nourish my mind, body and spirit—becoming more compassionate, happy, and balanced.*

Other clients also report that restorative, gentle yoga practice led to changes, including:

- *Slowly changing my thinking patterns to have more compassion for myself and others.*
- *Teaching me to love my body for the gift that it is, while giving me a new appreciation for the inner workings of my body—which truly is a miracle.*
- *Helping to manage stress (which often triggered binges) by slowing down and becoming more mindful.*

Partner Pose Classes

Partner yoga practice is dynamic and fulfilling. It is also complex and may not be suited for all clients (for example, clients with trauma from sexual or physical abuse). Already judging their bodies and obsessed about their appearance, clients with eating disorders are often skeptical of working with a partner. Hesitant at first, they are quiet and keep to themselves, resisting the suggestion that they engage with a classmate. However, after the instructor helps this initial discomfort and uneasiness subside, most find themselves laughing and making personal connections with one another.

I begin all partner work by asking the clients to sit in pairs on the floor, leaning against each other back to back. This allows the clients to make a physical connection without forced eye contact. Next, I ask them to become aware of their own breath. Then, I invite them to slowly notice their partner's breath. After her first partner yoga practice, Beth noted, "I was aware that my breath felt much quicker than my partner's. After a minute or two, I was able to slow my breath down to the pace of my partner's. It was like we were breathing together, and that was quite comforting."

I then ask the clients to begin to rock forward and back together. I do not instruct which way to lean first but, rather, encourage the pair to find their own unique rhythm. After these first two poses, I will ask what they noticed while practicing. Typical responses are:

- *At first I was scared about leaning on my partner. I was worried that I would crush her.*
- *What if I can't support him and he falls over?*
- *At first it's awkward to be so close to someone, but then you just breathe, relax and get out of your head. It's actually kind of fun to try something different, I even laughed a little, too.*

Other partner poses also foster connection, communication and harmony. These include, but are not limited to:

- Tree pose with partners standing side by side, holding hands as they reach for the sky.
- Warrior II with the outer edges of each partner's back foot touching as they reach in opposite directions.
- Boat pose with the partners' feet touching as they balance.

After a partner yoga practice, my client Emily shared:

I've never felt so supported and at the same time supportive of another person. We held each other up. I was even able to get out of my head and stopped judging myself. The eating disorder voice quieted down a bit, too, when I was able to just let go and realize that this was a team effort. I wasn't in charge and I didn't have to do anything "right."

Partner yoga can expand beyond poses for pairs. Once the class is calm and at ease with itself, I like to introduce group poses. My favorite is a group Warrior III. First, I teach everyone how to do this challenging balancing pose on their own, with no assistance or support from the group. When I ask for feedback after practicing Warrior III, clients have plenty to offer. As Jane put it: "I always feel off-balance in that pose. It's just really hard to stay centered."

This sets up my next variation, in which everyone in the group holds hands while practicing Warrior III. After trying it with the entire group's help, LaToya shared: "That was so much easier. I knew that I wasn't going to fall over this time." On the other hand, Becky reported: "I actually thought it was harder. I'm used to doing things on my own, so I didn't want to take responsibility if someone else fell because of me. And, I didn't want to take someone down with me."

This expression of contrasting views is common—and a fabulous opportunity for the instructor to discuss the issues arising within the group. Partner and group poses can foster discussion on the following topics:

• Being a supporter and being supported
• Independence and dependence
• Teamwork and collaboration.

Conclusion

The depth and diversity of the yoga practice make it an excellent modality for healing an eating disorder while facilitating the individual's unique journey to recovery. Whether focusing solely on one form of practice such as restorative, or practicing a variety of formats including a strong practice or a partner practice, yoga offers each client an opportunity to connect to the authentic self. The yoga practice becomes a direct pathway, leading the client back to the body that she had once rejected, feared and punished. From quietly witnessing the flow of breath to finding personal power in Warrior poses, yoga is a link between the head and the heart, the mind and the body.

Sharing the yoga practice with eating disorder clients is not always easy. I certainly meet resistance from time to time. Yet, witnessing such profound transformation makes any struggle completely worthwhile. I have experienced moments of deep appreciation and gratitude for yoga and my clients. It is a wonderful gift to gather my clients' voices and share their feedback about the ancient practice of yoga.

16 Athletes, Yoga and Eating Disorders

Jamie Silverstein

The Drug Test

I'm not a drug user, and never was. But I *have* failed a drug test. I failed it not because I was high or using; I failed it because I was suffering from anorexia nervosa.

Technically, I flunked because I wasn't producing urine with a high enough specific gravity to yield a valid result. Essentially, I was peeing water. That was the same night I became the US National Senior Ice Dancing silver medalist and I was offered a slot on the US World Team.

Sports governing bodies test athletes to prevent cheating, specifically the use of drugs or other supplements to enhance performance artificially. An official is assigned to the athlete who stays with you from the time you formally register for your test until the time the test is complete. The official monitors collection of the sample to ensure integrity. The official cannot leave your side until an adequate sample is accurately collected. No breaks. No privacy. No cheating or swapping.

On the ice, I always trained and competed fairly. But I was not fair with myself.

That night in the doping room, I felt frustrated. Already self-conscious about my eating disorder, I told myself that I *would* eat, that I *could* eat. Really. Not only for the urine test, but because I *deserved* some food after my medal-winning performance.

But, even after earning a silver medal at Nationals, I thought: "I already ate a cocoa-chocolate mix before free dance. And now, it's getting late. Of course, I can't eat any of the junky food available in the staging area. But I *am* going to have something to celebrate."

I ate some lettuce off a submarine sandwich.

Sometime after midnight, the arena had to close. It couldn't stay open simply because I couldn't pass my test. Still, I had yet to produce a useable urine sample. The doping was not over.

My doping agent thought she had been assigned to a healthy, vibrant, world-class athlete. Instead, she had to spend the night in a hotel with all 80 pounds of me. In the morning, I did finally pee a readable shade of yellow. I passed the doping screen and was invited onto the US World Team.

Athletes and Eating Disorders

To be successful, athletes are taught to perfect their bodies—usually by meeting an external ideal (petite ice dancer, skinny marathoner, bulky tight end). This often means learning to ignore or refute the body's physical signals for rest, pain relief, nourishment and other support. Ironically, embodiment is often lost in competitive physical sports. Instead, magical thinking develops: "If I can just ... [fill in the blank], I will win!"

Athletes in certain competitive sports regularly restrict water or food intake and/or train with injuries. Most sports teach you to master your physical body by consistently improving it. Even at young ages, athletes enter a never-ending quest to "be better." In pursuit of winning, coaches do not teach—and athletes do not learn—how to celebrate the body as it is. The disembodied drive to succeed produces famous sports mantras like: "no pain, no gain."

What happens when we ignore physical cues, and define our bodies as projects to be "perfected"? We undermine our experience of self and, more importantly, the practice of self-acceptance. It's virtually impossible to live a balanced, healthy life in such a state.

Hyper-vigilance over the body and disconnection from its needs were all but mandated for figure skaters when I competed. Eating disorders thrive in body vigilance and disconnection.

Both our athletic community and our wider society need to examine how regularly our culture celebrates and honors those who succeed at all costs—including a disconnection from the body and serious harm. For example, in the 1996 Olympics, gymnast Kerri Strug won fame by competing with damaged ankle tendons. "What courage!" people said. Football players still "play through" concussions despite evidence of long-term brain damage and early death, all while record numbers of us tune in to watch. In athletics, the achievement of the *body* becomes overly imbued with meaning, at the cost of the *person* inside it. And spectators cheer.

The clear message: winning demands that athletes punish their bodies and athletes respond because success is cultural currency; they want to feel virtuous, valuable, or at the very least, a part of the game. An analogous pseudo-logic pulses eerily through the eating disorder self.

It is no surprise then that high-performance sports—particularly those with an aesthetic or weight focus, like gymnastics, wrestling, diving, and figure skating—are plagued with broken bodies and disordered behaviors which remain (sometimes intentionally) overlooked or denied. Because many modern sports *require* an athlete to engage in some degree of self-harm (e.g., pushing past pain), the meta-culture of sports condones and normalizes disordered practices—and calls them "training."

Culturally defined expectations of what an athlete is (or should be) work to help an eating disorder thrive, and the competitors are not the only ones harmed. Our culture's parameters for athletes influence the rest of us.

Spectators don't want to see a "fat" (read: anything more than emaciated) figure skater at the Olympics and audiences don't want to see big ballerinas dance *Swan Lake*. In the end, these expectations come back to hurt all of us as they reinforce disordered perspectives elsewhere in society and even inform cultural ideals and icons.

Yoga and Athletics

Fortunately, there are alternative perspectives to approach and work with the body. When paired with athletic pursuits, yoga practice can teach athletes to locate themselves *within* their bodies. Over time, yoga's non-judgmental self-observation helps an athlete combat over-training, and disordered or excessive training regimes. In yoga, the athlete is confronted repeatedly with questions such as: "Where am I in my body? How do *I* feel? How can I offer myself compassion?" Yoga requires one to look in, rather than to perform out.

Simply, yoga encourages compassionate connection on an internal level between body, mind, and soul. This is categorically different from aesthetic or performance sports. In yoga, there is no score card and no panel of judges decides your fate. You practice; you don't perform.

Yoga and Embodiment

As a 15-year-old Midwestern girl, yoga had enough shock value to interest me ("is it a cult?"), and enough physicality to pass my mom's (and my eating disorder's) "things she is allowed to do with her free time" test. So I started practicing yoga. I never imagined that it would be a key to healing me later in life.

I took to yoga easily. As an elite athlete, I loved working my physical body. But I was also deeply connected to a disordered impulse that more was not only *better*; more was *necessary*. So, I did yoga classes nearly every day, but something else slowly started to happen. I began to experience and recognize the state of embodiment. As much as I *utilized* my body in figure skating, *I was not in my body*. Ironically, this is why I was both successful and sick.

Embodiment requires that you recognize that you are a whole person: a person with meaning, purpose, and life far beyond the current shape of your body or the size of its parts. Embodiment teaches us to recognize that we exist within a form (the body), but that our form is not our existence. Rather, our form is the vessel for the loves and lights of our life.

Only when we can abstract ourselves away from "being" a body and from seeing ourselves exclusively or primarily as only our body, can we cultivate a mutually beneficial, loving relationship with said body.

This was new for me. Yoga required that I be accountable to my own embodiment, and this accountability would soon become one of the greatest blessings in my life. Over time, I learned to see my body not as something to be managed or manipulated but as a vehicle to connection with myself and, ultimately, love. My skating career has come and gone; my time in yoga remains. In yoga, I practice meeting myself with genuine compassion, curiosity and love.

Embodiment and Eating Disorders

Like most eating disorder professionals, I believe you cannot heal the mind via the mind alone and you cannot fix the body via the body alone. Because yoga demands mindful integration, it complements traditional cognitive and behavioral therapies in concrete ways. Yoga promotes an embodied experience in which clients can practice actualizing important cognitive shifts necessary for recovery.

The practice of conscious embodiment is particularly relevant for people suffering with eating disorders. Embodiment teaches one to see *where* she or he is in an expressive body. That's radically opposed to the eating disorder construct, based on *what* one should change, limit, control or "fix" about her or his body.

In order to recover, eating disorder sufferers must accept an essential reality: the body is something to celebrate as a vehicle through which we may express ourselves, our love, and our connection to spirit. The body was never the problem; and painful manipulation or disconnection are not the solution. Yoga teaches us to feel this truth through its philosophy, embodied practice, and experience of connection.

Yoga takes time. It is often a subtle practice and the shifts in self-compassion and self-care can be hard to measure. Yoga acts as a conduit for self-acceptance, provided that one relates to oneself with curiosity and patience. With practice, clients re-establish trust with their senses, breath and ability to stay present. Yoga gives the practitioner real-time data on themselves and, consequently, real-life opportunities to regain meaning, strength and joy.

Over and over, I have seen how insights gained during yoga practice help people with eating disorders manage anxieties and practice self-compassion— ultimately learning to validate and appreciate their body and their needs. In this way, yoga brings self-acceptance on the mat, which ultimately transfers to other areas of our lives.

Yoga in Practice

When taught properly, yoga guides us to meet ourselves in the moment observing or beholding our thoughts—without judging those thoughts or shaming one's self. From there, one can encounter oneself from a higher, aware mind.

Yoga teaches us many ways to do this:

- We encounter the pulsation within our bodies.
- We train our mind to settle into the hypnotic transience of our breath.

- We notice that our thoughts are seldom new and we begin to act as our own personal witness.
- We begin to appreciate the difference between our thinking mind and our higher state awareness (witness consciousness).
- We understand that we are not our thoughts, even though we have a lot of them!
- We notice that our body has intelligence to communicate our needs astutely.
- We begin to recognize that we are something beyond our bones and our thoughts.

The yoga philosophy and Sanskrit teacher Manorama says: "One cannot be what one sees."[1] This concept is foundational in the treatment of eating disorders, because recovery requires that clients deeply accept the reality that they are so much more than a body—or their perceptions of the body's external appearance. Simply, to heal from an eating disorder, one must deeply recognize their worth far beyond the state of their body.

In yoga, when we talk about the body, we talk about our *relationship* with the body, a conversation which is also central to talk therapy for eating disorders. For one suffering from an eating disorder, it's vitally important to develop a set of tools to navigate this nuanced difference between *being* a body and *relating to* one's body.

People need to notice when their opinions of, and beliefs about, their body are filtering their experience of sensation. People with eating disorders especially need to re-engage actively with healthy relating and curiosity. When people can assess their body outside of their opinions or thought-loops, healing can take root.

Weaving Yoga Practice into Eating Disorders Treatment

In psychotherapy, people with eating disorders work on triggering thought patterns. Clients learn to listen for and challenge the "Eating Disorder" voice. Yoga can supplement this process by helping clients develop a witness consciousness while *simultaneously* experiencing physical counterpoints that go against the negative thoughts.

For example, if a client expresses negative thoughts about her belly, the yoga teacher can, in that moment, direct the client to experience the sweet feeling of taking a belly breath and the tactile comfort of lovingly placing her palms on her belly. Therapist and client can build upon these counterpoints, providing support to challenge destructive thought patterns.

For eating disorder thoughts like "My body is gross," I ask the client to notice *where* in the body this statement comes from. Is the person experiencing physical discomfort? Is this statement an opinion? Is this a catch-all for feeling heartache? Does it make the body act as a scapegoat or proxy for uncomfortable feelings?

Once clients have some insight into how their statements reflect deeper sensations or processes, I use prescriptive yoga practices to soothe, increase insight, and develop positive attributes to challenge eating disorder statements and beliefs.

One former client who managed her anxiety through eating disorder behaviors found help in very simple yoga exercises. For example, she practiced touching her fingertips to one another (hakini mudra) for focus as she did three-part-breathing. This did not cure her anxiety, but it taught her to witness and pause rather than resorting instantly to eating disorder symptoms. She also brought her developing insights into her talk therapy sessions.

We developed an ongoing plan to have yoga "run interference" with her anxiety. We made a deal: she agreed to set a timer and try her yogic plan for three minutes when she noticed her anxiety rising or when she was likely to encounter a trigger. If the yoga practices hadn't helped by the moment the timer sounded, she could try something else. The yoga worked.

The Role of Yoga Asana in Treatment

In yoga therapy groups for eating disorders, I teach clients to pay special attention to where and how physical sensation arises. I ask them to pay attention to any mental scripts that turn on as they encounter different aspects of their body. I encourage curiosity. The practice can be radical for clients whose feelings and emotions are distorted by stories they tell themselves.

For example, I often combine reflection and asana, beginning a group by giving clients a simple figure outline. I invite them to fill out the sheet with the thoughts, emotions, and/or personal stories they place on their bodies, paying mind to *where* they locate them. I then ask clients to review their work for a few moments, noticing areas that bring up particularly charged responses.

Next, we practice a slow asana flow with special attention on mindfulness and calming breath work (pranayama). When appropriate, I encourage clients to work with eyes shut. Sometimes, carefully, I use therapeutic touch. We finish with a full-body meditation offering gratitude and loving-kindness to each part of the body. With a hand on the heart, we repeat the phrase: "Dear body, I love you."

After practice, we return to the figure outlines. This time I instruct clients to inscribe what they remember about the *experience* of their bodies during the asana and meditation. The changes are profound. When clients can see how their experience *within* their body is so drastically different to their opinion of their body, they are better able to refute their eating disorder statements. This teaches clients the value of *coming back to mindfulness* as a tool to combat their thoughts.

In treatment, clients learn *where* their emotions live and *how* their body responds. Clients learn to witness their thoughts and how their thoughts can instigate emotions. With practice, a client develops the mindfulness to separate her or his authentic experience from the momentary wave of an emotion or thought. Empowerment and freedom come from being able to have thoughts and feelings without becoming overwhelmed by them, having to act on them, or struggling to get rid of them.

This is precisely how yoga works to serve eating disorder recovery. Yoga helps clients stay with, breathe through and navigate reactions without engaging in eating disorder behaviors to cope—providing grounded access to the physical and emotional self.

Action vs Reaction in Yoga

In yoga practice, a person learns to *respond* rather than react by investigating and experiencing oneself as an agent—a person who chooses. Yoga is a practice of self-agency, learning to break away from conditioned, habitual reactions.

Yoga provides a primer for people to encounter and understand their natural waves of thoughts and feelings, without forfeiting their sense of "I" to those momentary sensations. This is particularly relevant for those suffering with eating disorders. They gain compassion and healing as they learn: "I am not my body, I am the energy which moves it; I am not my thoughts, I am the force which directs them."

Simultaneously, yoga practice helps us find our spirit or internal wisdom. When clients become sensitized to their own energy, they learn to observe and study the patterns that underlie their reactions. Yoga provides space to learn that feelings or opinions do not have to lead to behavior. Yoga encourages people to engage *actively* in all of their experience—reaction, response, pleasure, distress, etc.—from a conscious, curious, mindful space.

In the process of recovery, talk therapy and yoga both help clients cultivate consciousness around responding vs reacting, while learning explicit skills for distress tolerance, mindfulness, awareness, and healthful agency. These experiences build compassion, self-trust, and, healing.

Meeting Needs in a Healthy Way

It is important for eating-disorder clients to recognize underlying needs that contribute to their dysfunctional behaviors, and learn to replace those behaviors with ones that meet their needs in a healthy way.

Yoga creates a safe environment to begin a process of curiosity and self-discovery. During yoga, clients learn a new embodied self-dialogue much different and healthier than their eating disorder chatter. Yoga may not change a client's thoughts, but it does teach how to observe the whirling mind (chitta vrittis) with compassion. As we learn to watch the movements of the mind, we become aware of our traps and incomplete (read: opinion-driven) translations of our experiences.

Yoga's practice of embodiment and self-witnessed experience was central to my recovery. It was only when I learned to ask: "Is that thought based in physical experience right now?" and "What is this impulse or feeling really about?" that I began to recognize the value of understanding my thought patterns and urges. By training myself to stay with experience without engaging in symptoms, I could handle what arrived. I began to understand on a deep level that symptomatic behaviors might be *a* choice but they were not my *only* choice. Through the steadiness of asana, I began to understand that I could choose what I made out of events and how I reacted or responded to them.

Yoga and the Self

Yoga practices help a person hold the space for an ever-developing relationship with the self. With dedicated practice, we become a witness and a loving friend to all aspects of ourselves—including our body.

Like many others with eating disorders, I evaluated myself against my perception of how others judged me, and I believed those perceptions. Attention from others signified acceptance; athletic prowess would keep me loved and safe. At the same time, I sensed a longing to challenge my beliefs, which I intrinsically knew were unfair and harmful. I did not want to be loved because of my successes. But I had not yet learned that I was intrinsically lovable. To heal, I needed an alternative way of seeing *me*. I needed to encounter myself beyond the physical result of what I did or didn't do.

One way to begin to befriend ourselves is by learning how to be vulnerable. This means admitting our imperfection, sharing our truth, and accepting where we are. Yoga can facilitate this acceptance through the practice of being exactly where one is, in terms of the ability to do a pose or sit with uncomfortable feelings.

In my groups, I encourage clients to love the tender parts of themselves without shame, judgment or critique. We laugh at our misguided minds and refute our tendency to practice "comparison-asana." I teach clients how to observe breath and sensation in a yoga framework which is radically different from their critical, disparaging eating disorder narrative. This helps clients learn to listen to themselves and practice self-acceptance and compassion.

Perspectives from Recovery

Eating disorders have a way of re-patterning the brain into mazes of self-induced guilt and shame. My disordered mind ran me in circles, demanding that I see each bite of food and every misstep as an episode in the story of being unlovable as I was. I felt that I was fundamentally damaged and to blame for everything. That was my story, but, thankfully, not my destiny. I am recovered. This took reevaluation. This took love. This took me accepting and valuing me, as is.

Early on in my yoga practice, a teacher encouraged me to take a break from the physical movement so that I could listen to the hum of my body; not my mind, my body. This was a pivotal moment in my relationship to myself: *there was something within me to hear.*

Yoga encouraged me to delve *into* this knowledge, not distance myself from it the way my athletics and eating disorder did. This perspective was stunning. Coupled with the loving encouragement of teachers and fellow students, I began to believe there was an alternative way of feeling and being in relationship with my body and myself.

Yoga taught me about myself *within* the context of my form. It gave me space and tools to start observing *how* I related with myself and my body, instead of my identity being dependent on how my body performed at the next competition.

Yoga gave me a radically different physical experience: embodied, playful movement. Because I was athletic, physical yoga practices provided a profoundly translatable counterpoint that I hadn't encountered previously.

It took years of practice, petulance and conditional promises before I really believed what so many already know: we are inherently lovable. Yoga teaches that we are love and everything else is just chatter which draws us away.

This is why I love yoga and always make room for it. I need a place to land within myself. This does not mean that I obsessively practice asana every day. Obsessive asana is not yoga. Instead, my yoga practice involves seeing myself and my actions through the lens of patience and love on the mat, in meditation and when stuck in traffic. I practice breathing, listening and curiosity. I recognize my humanity as a starting point, not a folly. I've learned to trust myself.

Through this practice, I *have* been transformed. I learned to live *within* my body, not be the enforcer of it. From within my body, I can objectively see my form and offer it tenderness. This is genuine tenderness, the kind I easily offer to my friends and my beloved. I consider this the best type of victory.

Today, all of me knows that it is not my body's responsibility to prove my worth.

In fact, it never was.

Note

1 See http://sanskritstudies.org/about/manorama (retrieved June 22, 2015).

Part 4

Integrating Yoga in Eating Disorder Treatment Programs

17 Opening the Door to Yoga in Treatment: Guidance and Guidelines

Carolyn Costin

Yoga as a component of eating disorder treatment is rewarding *and* challenging. Clients with eating disorders share many similarities *and* they each struggle in their own individual ways. Yoga teachers working with eating disorders will encounter familiar issues seen with other students but there are some unique considerations when working with this population.

As discussed earlier in this book, yoga was incorporated into the first Monte Nido residential treatment center and, due to its success, remains an integral part of all our residential and day treatment programs. The following information and guidelines are provided in hopes that others can benefit from our experience.

Client Participation

Since all our clients, then and now, are medically cleared for outings and other activities during residential treatment, we offer appropriate yoga experiences to most clients. We developed three levels of participation, Floor Yoga, Level 1 and Level 2. Most clients start on Floor Yoga or Level 1. Floor Yoga is used for clients who are very underweight or there is some other reason why the staff feels the client should not participate in the slightly more active Level 1.

In Floor Yoga clients do gentle stretches while lying on their mats. It is easy to incorporate simple restorative postures and use bolsters to move the Floor yogis through a series of supported reclining poses somewhat similar to Level 1 and 2 poses. This helps all clients feel connected, even if they are on different levels. For example, a teacher may use ardha chandrasana with Level 2 clients, trikonasana with Level 1, and a supported supta padanagusthasna with the clients on Floor level. Our teachers also move Floor clients through several different supported shapes during the course of the class, so they don't feel neglected or forgotten while the Level 1 and Level 2 students are moving more actively.

For Level 1 yoga, we decided on a gentle flow which includes sitting or kneeling poses, relatively simple standing poses and modified versions of more difficult poses. We designed Level 2 yoga with more standing poses, a quicker flow and the opportunity to try more challenging poses. When a client makes appropriate progress (e.g. weight gain, following the meal plan, and other goals specific to each individual), they can request on their weekly treatment contract to move to a higher level in the overall program and in yoga class.

The Yoga Teacher's Knowledge, Flexibility and Experience

Although our first teacher, Lauren Peterson, had taught classes of varying ability, none had participants as varied as those in residential treatment. Clients with extremely low weights, extremely high weights, multiple diagnoses and various levels of motivation were in class together. Through trial and error Lauren became comfortable dealing with all varieties of eating disorder clients, teaching students with widely varying levels of willingness and ability. Lauren learned and taught her successors that the yoga teacher must be prepared, flexible and attentive; consistently paying attention to all clients and adjusting things quickly and accordingly. In a single class, teachers might need to provide a variety of alternatives, stop some clients from pushing too far or too fast, and encourage others to make at least a minimal attempt at something.

Dealing with Emotions

Emotional stuff comes up in yoga. Emotions can be triggered by a pose, closing one's eyes, being silent, or experiencing what it feels like to be in one's body. Touching can bring tears of relief to one client, while causing another to stiffen and panic. Clients with eating disorders can be especially sensitive about their bodies. Some have suffered abuse or trauma. Yoga teachers often "adjust" clients in poses without thinking. We believe it is important to refrain from adjusting clients until a well understood sense of trust and safety has been established and the client has given permission for the teacher to do so. There are those who advise never adjusting another person in a pose.[1] However, some clients experience a profound sense of acceptance, relief and healing with a simple hand on the back or touch on the head.[2]

Teachers need to ask clients regularly to comment on what sensations, thoughts and feelings are coming up—and incorporate the feedback. At times one client might need to simply rest in child's pose or sit comfortably while others continue. It is important to pass these lessons on to any new yoga teachers or yoga therapists hired.[3]

Terminology

Yoga teachers must understand and agree to use the philosophy, modalities and terminology other treatment provider(s) are using with the client(s), so that the yoga reinforces and does not conflict. Additionally, language carries meaning and yoga teachers need to be thoughtful regarding the words they use. For example, at Monte Nido we believe clients can be fully "recovered" from their eating disorder thus it is important that our yoga teachers don't tell the clients they will always be "recovering."

Teachers should avoid or be careful with seemingly innocent words and phrases, such as "firm," "lean," or "full belly." These words have different connotations for people with eating disorders, and can easily trigger destructive thoughts, feelings and symptoms. Words and phrases need to be chosen wisely and thoughtfully. Clients should occasionally be asked how they are experiencing the class or if they are "triggered" by anything.

The Yoga Teacher is an Integral Part of the Team

We learned early on that the yoga teacher needs to be an important part of the whole team, participating in staff meetings and/or using other ways to share feedback with the rest of the staff. The yoga teacher and the rest of the client's treatment team are beholden to each other on many levels. Communication between all parties is key in making yoga a truly integrated part of treatment, rather than just a class or two taken during the week and/or a means of exercise. The yoga teacher's ability to facilitate the treatment team's goals will depend on the level and quality of communication.

Prior to class yoga teachers should check in with the therapist, staff, or clinical director to discuss any particular issues they need to pay attention to or address. The yoga teachers should also give feedback to the client's therapist, clinical director, or in staff meetings. Progress notes should also be made in the client's medical record.

Yoga Assisting with the Therapy and Treatment Goals

The value of yoga's integration becomes evident when yoga teachers incorporate into their classes what the clients are working on in therapy groups and/or individual sessions. Working together, the team and yoga teacher can come up with specific ways yoga can assist specific goals. For example, yoga teachers can teach anxious clients anti-anxiety breathing techniques to use before meals, during group, or before bed. The teacher should check in with the staff about any themes or milieu issues such as self-compassion or comparison, and choose readings from yoga teachings which teach about these concepts. Reading or listening to passages on self-compassion combined with practicing specific poses that help exemplify it, facilitates embodiment of the concept.[4] Some clients might ask for help with specific issues such as the ability to focus better or improve their digestion. Yoga teachers can help by prescribing specific poses or sequences that might be beneficial. Clients recognize the benefits:

> *Yoga surprisingly helped my headaches which allowed me to better participate in the rest of treatment.*

Learning breathing exercises in yoga changed my relationship to therapy. I was able to calm down during sessions and groups in a way I had never known before.

Stay Away from Promoting Dietary Preferences or Advice

It is important for yoga teachers working with eating disorders to refrain from promoting or even discussing any kind of food preferences like vegetarianism, veganism, periodic fasting, or juice cleanses. While these practices might be good for some people, they can be problematic and even dangerous for those with eating disorders. Eating disorder clients must avoid extremes, learn to restrict less, fear food less, eat enough, and not use food to cope. Balance is the key. Many eating disorder clients will take concepts like "fasting," "organic," or "vegetarian" to extremes, while others will feel guilty and humiliated for not following such food rules and restrictions.

I have seen damage done by healthy, well-meaning yoga teachers and by teachers who were unwell and out of balance themselves. This point was driven home by a particularly disturbing incident involving a former client with a long history of anorexia and severe anemia. She became a vegetarian during her eating disorder and it took a long time to convince her she needed to eat red meat for her particular health needs. During treatment she began eating meat again, gained weight, and started menstruating. She also became very fond of yoga and found it to be extremely helpful in her recovery. In fact she became inspired to become a yoga teacher.

During a weekend away at her teacher training, she and the fellow students in her class were forced to watch a video of animal slaughters in order to convince them to become vegans. She suffered a huge setback. Not only was she traumatized and unable to bring herself to continue to eat meat, she started suffering again from panic attacks that had subsided a year earlier. This event caused a significant relapse in her recovery and well-being. Eventually she got back on track with her eating but is still suffering from anxiety even at the thought of going back to yoga.

Unless it is simply to welcome the idea of needing to eat freely and nourish one's body, I implore yoga teachers working with the eating disorder population to stay away from the topic of food.

Client Resistance

Occasionally there are clients who resist yoga. If yoga is required some clients might resent being told they "have to go." Others might go to class but be unwilling to accept direction or follow instructions. Yoga teachers will likely be unfamiliar with these dynamics since private lessons and classes at yoga studios are not compulsory and only willing students show up. Lauren needed guidance in how best to handle clients in the treatment setting who did not participate or who outright disrupted a class. We worked out various strategies for dealing with these issues and always had a therapist available. All yoga teachers need direction and support from the team on how to handle this and other issues that might arise.

Learning to Let Go

While yoga brought positive results to the vast majority of our eating disorder clients, we have learned with some disappointment and dismay that certain people will simply not take to yoga. Even after carefully trying many paths and methods, some clients say they do not like it, it does not "work" for them, or it makes them feel worse. These problems are often a matter of timing, teacher, or environment—but sometimes changing these factors does not help.

Yoga cannot be forced on anyone. Clients at our programs who don't want to *do* yoga are still asked to attend the class. However, they can choose to sit quietly or lie down on the floor, just being there. When this happens, both the client and we are given an opportunity to practice the yoga of acceptance and letting go.

Notes

1 See Chapter 4.
2 See Chapter 7.
3 See Chapter 9.
4 See Chapters 13 and 14.

18 How Yoga Teachers Can Incorporate Yoga into Eating Disorder Treatment

Lisa Diers

Suppose you are a psychologist, yoga teacher, dietitian, yoga therapist, or executive who wants to bring yoga into an existing eating disorders treatment program. Here are just a few questions you'll need to consider:

- Why *would* we integrate yoga with the other modalities we use?
- How *do* we integrate yoga with other modalities we use?
- How do we persuade colleagues and decision-makers of yoga's benefits?
- How do we find the space, schedule and resources for it?
- How can we help staff understand the role and the potential benefits for:
  - group therapy
  - individual therapy
  - meal time/meal time management
  - established programs, such as Intensive Outpatient, Residential, Partial Hospitalization, Family Support, etc.
- How can we make it last?
- Does our program have to "see yoga in everything" it does from now on?

Drawing on a case study of The Emily Program (TEP) for eating disorders, this chapter discusses specific strategies to help treatment professionals start integrating yoga and keep it as a vibrant element of treatment and recovery. I hope to help those curious or nervous about yoga in treatment to better understand the fears—and experience the benefits. I invite you to imagine the possibilities for integration, and the fire that they can ignite within you!

In 2008, when I was a registered dietitian and certified yoga teacher, The Emily Program launched a "Yoga and Body Image" group in an unused warehouse space with wires hanging from an unfinished ceiling.

Seven years later, TEP had more than 40 yoga groups a week and each facility has at least one dedicated yoga room where yoga teachers work alongside clients of every diagnosis and in conjunction with other treatment modalities.

Yoga and Treatment

I used to tell clients that "In recovery, the only way out is through." Now I firmly believe that the only way out is *in*—into reconnection with the body and the genuine self and out of the abyss of the disorder.

Eating disorders bring a profound disconnection from body, creating a perfect emotional storm of fear, anger, anxiety, frustration, resistance, flashbacks and more. On the other hand, both food and yoga bring embodiment. In fact, they require embodiment. Yoga provides a way to build the connection between mind, body and spirit.

Yoga is like a well-equipped Range Rover®, excellent for entering and exploring the jungle of eating disorders. More than that, yoga strengthens one's internal navigation system to catch, challenge and change destructive ways of thinking and reacting.

With the right teaching approach, yoga is a powerful recovery force in multidisciplinary treatment. In fact, yoga and traditional eating disorder treatment mirror each other in ways that you might not recognize at first glance. For example, as a dietitian, I facilitate the connection with the body by encouraging clients to nourish its physical needs. As a yoga teacher, I facilitate the nurturance of emotional, mind-body and soul connections.

In both roles, I am a teacher and also a student, living by the principles I learned while becoming a Registered Dietitian:

- I learn from my clients how to guide, direct, lead and follow.
- I am a truth seeker, a "seer" of others' true self. I am honest, clear, and dependable. I won't abandon the client no matter how rough it gets.
- I am firm, yet compassionate. My clients' appreciation and affection are not required for me to be effective. Their fear is strong; working together, we are stronger.
- I listen, create a structure, provide options, and help the client set their own course.
- I am a scientist. I track trends, notice patterns, and share the data with my client without judgment. We then work together to make changes and incorporate new patterns.
- I am invested in their recovery and how it looks for them. I do not judge.
- I am curious. Not furious. I understand that my clients have difficulty trusting me.
- The truth is scary to face. It's not always easy to tell someone what they need. But it's what they trust me to do.
- I treat others how I would want to be treated.
- I respect my clients. They are the strongest people I know.

When integrating yoga into treatment, it's important to recognize—and communicate—the parallels between the methods and goals of yoga, psychotherapy, nutrition, medicine, and other elements of client care.

Adapting to Eating Disorder Dynamics

When management of yoga passed to me, I noticed that clients discussed anything and everything in class except eating disorders or body issues.

I realized we needed a consistent group norm. Clients are used to living with the structure which their eating disorder provides. We can't expect them to enter into a new, unfamiliar territory without clear guidelines. So I created the group norm of "discussing *only* what comes up in your body during today's yoga class." No talk about meal plans, symptoms, movies, books, or other things distracting from the experience.

Yoga clients take on this norm with surprising ease. They support and reinforce it with one another, creating an atmosphere of a peer-led group, while teachers lead from behind.

Yoga teachers and yoga therapists need to develop group skills, and learn how to create safety and non-judgment. They need to learn how best to:

- Remain silent
- Provide commentary
- Let the group lead itself
- Redirect the group and/or individuals
- Observe an experience unfolding
- Offer support, without interrupting the often-difficult healing process

Yoga teachers must work from a non-reactive stance, providing clients with a living, breathing and moving counterpoint to the highly reactive state of their eating disorder. We are mirrors to the experience, keeping a calm, professional, compassionate demeanor. We remain guides and witnesses, confident that we can be in the presence of the eating disorder self without surrendering to it.

We give clients concrete data for their efforts. The teacher speaks to or asks about specific physical or emotional themes as they relate to the class. Success means both teacher and therapist are partners in the client's exploration of these experiences.

Communicating and Selling the Benefits of Incorporating Yoga

Through client feedback and observations, yoga's healing benefits became apparent to therapists and teachers leading the groups. But other colleagues didn't always understand the value. In addition to leading the groups (and doing our other jobs), we needed to educate the agency's stakeholders: clients, therapists, dietitians, physicians, administrators and other staff.

We began by seizing opportunities. For instance, I offered to teach yoga when new or existing groups needed coverage. This nurtured relationships with staff and clients at multiple locations and created openness to yoga as a treatment tool.

If you want to add yoga to a current program you need to communicate intent and "sell" your "product." For instance, you cannot expect an executive to green light yoga because you are passionate about yoga's healing capabilities. Remember that each manager, therapist, dietitian, or physician is just as passionate about their treatment center, specific discipline and the clients they serve. They are going to be understandably protective and ask some tough questions.

Take the time to learn about the agency and the multi-disciplinary team who do this work every day. Try to anticipate their questions. What might the therapist, dietitian, or physician want to know about yoga? How might yoga affect the work they do with their clients? How can you help them anticipate the challenges and maximize the benefits? Share a copy of this book to educate them.

Eating disorders are multifaceted problems unique to each person and the illness is a master of disguise. You can't assume you know it all. Approach each client and colleague with clarity of intent and a beginner's mind: willing to ask, listen and learn.

Take the time to dig deep and ask *yourself* tough and important questions:

- What is my intention?
- What do I know and not know about eating disorders? Who will I consult with and learn from?
- How can I do no harm?
- Does what I want to offer fit into the company's overall mission and vision? My own?
- Can I set aside my own ego and do what needs to be done? Can I welcome the challenging questions as opportunities to grow?
- Can I modify my approach to meet the key decision makers where they are, not where I think they should be?
- Can I see situations through the multidisciplinary team's eyes?
- Can I communicate effectively?
- If I were a client, what kind of experience would I want to have? What might I be nervous about or want to understand?
- If I were an executive, what might I care about?

Anticipate rejection; if you get it, be curious, not furious. If there is resistance, ask for an explanation. How can you educate? Can you offer a free class by coming to them or having them come to your studio? Can they take 10 minutes for you to give them a yoga experience? Take advice and guidance from concerned colleagues.

Too Much Too Soon: A Lesson in Backing Off

Once yoga started taking off at TEP, I put a lot of energy into getting the news out to our team through any and every communication channel.

Looking back, it may have been a bit obnoxious for a dietitian to add information about yoga (especially staff yoga) to every one of her "all staff" emails or repeatedly distribute flyers in staff mail boxes, offices and meetings. I saw the potential and it was burning a fire in me. But not everyone was ready for my intensity.

Fortunately, a dear colleague and mentor called and said: "You need to back off of the yoga emails."

"Really? Why?" I asked.

"Other people are getting annoyed."

Crap! I'd just hit send on another yoga-related email!

I felt bad, but could see it from another perspective. I backed off but kept my passion. To spread yoga agency-wide, I had to adjust my pace and meet key decision makers where they were. This was a lesson in patience and timing (a yoga lesson itself). Leaders and decision makers ultimately connected with the passion I felt, when I wasn't shoving it in their face!

I was invited to do yoga presentations during staff meetings, in-service trainings and new staff orientations. We discussed integrating yoga with nutrition, art therapy, music therapy and massage. We began offering regular yoga sessions for staff—to ease stress and build community. We did "guest" yoga presentations and classes for the friends and family groups. This strategy of measured and mindful exposure worked beautifully.

Soon, colleagues were asking us how to integrate yoga into their work. University of Minnesota researchers wanted our data to study the impact of yoga on eating disorders. Demand for classes and groups continued to skyrocket.

Meanwhile, I continued to listen very closely to fellow treatment providers who seemed resistant to yoga. I intentionally found ways to ally with them while working as a myth buster, educator and collaborator.

Yoga for EveryBODY!

One day at an outpatient program, I met several clients who were particularly nervous about participating. One was paraplegic and questioned her ability to do yoga. Another feared she was not flexible enough. A third was convinced that her large body size would be an obstacle to movement. I discussed their fears and explained why we do yoga in treatment.

I explained how yoga cultivates body awareness, acceptance and appreciation. We start with simple ways to connect and listen to the messages the body has for us. We practice being curious about those messages; after all, they are just information. We have a choice about what to "do" with the information. I said that TEP yoga teachers always explain what to expect in detail (what to wear, shoes on or off, props, my role, their role, ways to do adaptive yoga, where the bathroom is, etc.). Plus, yoga is fun.

I led them through a five-minute sampler of uncomplicated asanas they could do while standing or sitting. During each pose, we explored the experience of noticing one's body and taking up space. I also invited the clients to stay in a pose "for three seconds longer than you think you can." Next, I asked: "What else can you do that you don't think you can do?" Finally, I explained how, even in these simplest activities, "yoga is *already* creating an opportunity to appreciate your body for what it can do, versus what it looks like."

Eventually, clients of every ability, shape and diagnosis were seeing yoga for what it could be for them. Not what it should be. There is no "should" in yoga.

Soon our work was referred to as "Yoga for EveryBODY." The yoga was speaking for itself through the clients. Yoga class became as valuable as any group or meal.

Remember that yoga is only a tool. In any mental health setting, its power works in conjunction with the other multidisciplinary approaches in the treatment toolbox. Yoga is an option. It may not be the way for everyone.

Qualities of Successful Groups

Yoga teachers must remember that we are competing with a loud and powerful eating disorder voice. Much of what we say is not heard at all, not heard fully, or else heard in a way that supports old beliefs. When training new yoga instructors, I ask clients in my yoga group to start talking with each other while I am teaching. This helps new teachers to grasp the intense eating disorder voice which clients must manage while trying to move in a yoga class—and drives home the challenge of teaching in this setting.

In order to create a safe space that clients can trust, the teacher must honestly, calmly and regularly name eating disorder behaviors—without judgment. In yoga, you and your client have a rare opportunity to "see" the illness in action—to witness the eating disorder embodied. Identifying the behaviors during yoga can help the client recognize the connection between themselves and their disorder, and begin separating the two. Yoga provides clients with methods to "read" how their emotional barometers respond to life's challenges. It also embodies the idea that they have choice—including the choice to cope and self-soothe in a way that works best for them.

Trust develops by maintaining confidentiality in yoga groups and classes. Nothing leaves the safety of the yoga room unless it is yours and you take it with you. Not honoring this commitment is grounds for discharge from the group.

We encourage teachers to be clear, concise, confident, and curious, setting an example for the clients to follow. Start with the basics and build. Our clients are rediscovering and repairing their relationship to their bodies. Through yoga movement, clients re-pattern their bodies' responses and lay down new neuro-pathways.

Too many words can confuse and distract clients, reinforcing the old familiar disordered voice and patterns. Pay attention to how your students hear your words and adjust your language accordingly. Don't get caught up in your own practice. Your job in these moments is to teach and observe the results.

You'll begin to notice trends. I find that adolescents prefer more movement, "fun" poses, laughter and music. Adults are more drawn to reflection, grounding and centering. Clients with anorexia and/or bulimia respond well to intentional linking of breath and movement. Clients with binge eating disorder or compulsive overeating need more reassurance and practice with letting go of judgment. But there is more commonality than difference among diagnoses. Across the board, you're likely to notice manifestations of avoidance, distraction, comparisons and anxiety.

Yoga in Therapeutic Meals

Dietitians and therapists eat with TEP clients at every meal—a co-facilitation that is challenging, transformative and reverent. During therapeutic meals, we create a safe space where clients can connect to their eating disorder coping strategies. They can explore their experience with curiosity about thoughts, feelings and behaviors.

This makes mealtime fertile territory for integrating yoga's goal of facilitating observer mind. Guidelines for integrating yoga at meals:

- Schedule yoga immediately before meals and snacks
- Practice simple breathing before meal time
- Have clients do a favorite pose before the meal
- Bring awareness to body language while waiting for the meal
- Encourage breathing and joking to relieve meal-related tension
- Guided Centering before and halfway through meal time
- Remove shoes and keep feet on the floor throughout the meal
- Use yoga movements, e.g., before meals to reduce anxiety and after to aid digestion

These guidelines influence the eating environment, making it easier to gather information and make observations about mood, tension, fidgeting, food manipulation and other behaviors. At the table anxious clients can be asked to relax their shoulders, stop shaking, and deepen their breath—and then asked: "Did any of those body adjustments help calm you or adjust your thoughts?"

Adapting to Treatment Climate, Diagnosis, and Physical Ability

Yoga teachers have to expect the unexpected when they teach eating disorder clients. Go into class with a plan, and be ready to change it. You may not know what happened in the process group the clients just finished or what they might be anticipating for the next event in their day. So, be prepared for struggles to unfold on the mat.

Our initial yoga and Body Image group was the first "mixed diagnosis" group at our agency. As yoga helped peel back the outer layers, and helped uncover the amazing similarities among the clients with varying diagnoses.

Working with clients at their level is important. This can be difficult when teaching people with every type of experience, ability, diagnosis, age and body state. The less we make someone's difference stand out, the more comfortable everyone will feel.

The following instructions will help:

- Before class, orient students to props and/or adaptations they may need.
- Continuously remind clients, "there is no wrong or right way to do yoga." Adapt the posture to fit the student, NOT the student to the posture.
- Encourage all clients to try poses, and do what feels best for them.
- Use the power of your words to guide the class. E.g., teach Sun Salutations in a way that is simultaneously accessible to every person practicing from a chair, a mat, or the wall.
- Refrain from judgment or comparison of clients who can only work from an adaptive foundation (such as a chair).
- Offer your support from a stance of curiosity, not correction.
- Notice and acknowledge patterns and make suggestions.
- Name and calmly challenge resistance. If a client refuses, ask:

  - Can you tell me Why?
  - What is your intention in this moment?
  - What have you done in the past when you felt this way?
  - What would be helpful now?
  - What would you like to do instead and why?

Encourage clients to try at least three poses in each session. If clients need to rest in savasana, even for long periods of the class, honor that choice. Congratulate clients for honoring their body and what it needs.

The clients often provide us with feedback on postures, sequences, and language. We find this valuable in improving our effectiveness. For example, I taught ustrasana (Camel pose) in every class, verbally encouraging students to "get something off your chest."

One day a client who struggled with gender identity approached me after class and said: "Lisa, every time you say 'get something off your chest,' all I think about is getting rid of my disgusting breasts!" She loved ustrasana, but wished I would use different language. I thanked her for sharing this perspective, which had not occurred to me. We discussed ideas, and agreed that saying "let something go" instead is much better.

This was a great lesson in listening and underlined the value of creating an environment where clients learn to trust that they can share their experience and trust we will work together to find a solution.

Based on our yoga for eating disorder treatment study, we now offer yoga five days a week in residential treatment and are increasing its frequency in outpatient programming. We consider yoga to be a core eating disorder treatment modality.

Finding Quality Teachers

In an environment of yoga studios dedicated to aerobics, toning and looking good, it's a major challenge to find yoga teachers who understand puzzling eating disorders—and who will facilitate healing. The challenge is similar to finding eating disorder-sensitive dietitians in a weight-loss world.

I look for teachers who are intuitive, compassionate and prepared to be disliked or unappreciated. Like other treatment professionals, yoga teachers must expect resistance while simultaneously maintaining respect, compassion and good intentions toward the client. An effective yoga teacher cares about the client and can differentiate between the person and the products of their eating disorder. Even when interactions are rough and the symptoms complex, we have to stay with the reality that the person is not their disorder—and that struggle is part of recovery.

Both veteran and new teachers say that adopting new language and attitudes is the most challenging part of working in the treatment setting. It can take six months to a year for teachers to feel confident about the work.

If a candidate has potential, we usually conduct three interviews, including one where they show us how they teach. We ask potential teachers a series of essential questions, including:

- Why do you want to work in eating disorders treatment?
- What is your experience working in a treatment or mental health setting? If none, describe how you think your personality traits and teaching style would fit in our setting.
- What is your yogic philosophy?
- What is your food philosophy?
- How do you feel about eating meals with clients?
- Give an example of a difficult situation and how you approached it.
- What is your experience working with a team?
- What kind of communicator are you?
- Explain a time when you had to modify your class to meet the needs of a client. How did you know modification was needed?
- What is your self-care practice?
- Sometimes this work is sad when we witness our clients struggle. As a teacher it is important not to "fix the emotional pain." Rather, we have compassion, but also remember that the learning happens through the struggle. Can you speak to this?
- Explain how you handle multitasking.
- Without demonstrating, instruct me through a sun salutation.

- In treatment, clients frequently compare or critique a yoga teacher's body, as they struggle with their own reality. How do you imagine handling body judgments and comparisons directed (verbally and nonverbally) toward you or other clients?

Experience taught us not to settle. Current teachers will find ways to cover classes ourselves before hiring a "second best" new teacher who can't adequately impart the necessary philosophy.

Graduates of a registered program have an advantage, but the teaching tells it all. We have the candidate teach to two staff members, preferably another yoga teacher and a therapist. If you are the interviewer, think like a client when you are in the interview and during the "interview" class. If you feel confused, rushed, or uncomfortable, chances are good that clients will feel the same.

Connection with Colleagues

If something significant happens in yoga, the teacher communicates it to dietitians and/or therapists right after class. We work openly and directly with our partners in treatment, learning from them and sharing with them. We adapt yoga class to the needs and issues arising for clients—and encourage clients to discuss their yoga practice openly in group and individual therapy. We are now piloting one-on-one yoga consultations to meet the needs of clients, like those with severe trauma, who struggle in class settings.

One day, clients came to my class visibly angry over an incident in the process group prior to yoga. The upset carried into and disrupted class. So, I put aside my agenda and sat everyone in a circle for some tough love. I described what I was seeing: they wanted to continue the drama of the process group and not do yoga.

"This is exactly why we do yoga here," I said. "This is an opportunity to 'hold both' your anger and your yoga." We decided the best thing to do was to try holding the emotion while moving ahead with the yoga tasks at hand. The movement and breath work demonstrated concretely that the emotional mind only has as much power as we give it; we have choices!

Near the end of class, I looped back around to the experience and noted the different energy in the room. The participants had ridden out the emotional wave through yoga—and they knew it. I invited them to imagine the possibilities for self-regulation off the yoga mat! Yoga is like any other part of treatment: catch it, challenge it and decide to change it.

When the class was over, I made sure to check in with the process group therapist, and we collaborated in the following weeks to reinforce one another's efforts.

Communicate your observations to colleagues. Discuss what you see, and what you imagine seeing next. Share your knowledge about what yoga can do—and what yogis have known for thousands of years.

Connection with Clients

In eating disorders treatment, yoga helps clients connect. That connection is not easy and not always enjoyable. Therefore, we must educate our students on the why of yoga—especially why we ask them to practice elements of yoga in treatment.

We must prove to clients that we are allied with them, on the same team, giving and expecting honesty, demonstrating that they can trust us and that we will trust them. Be curious, name the challenges and connect with the victories. This leads to adaptability and flexibility for teacher and students.

We invite the process to unfold before us. We help guide clients through their inevitable moments of distress, showing them how to see distress as information. Rather than avoid difficulty, we intentionally and openly do the thing (pose, sequence, breathing) that clients don't want to do. If any idea or situation brings up an emotional charge, we value its exploration and avoid avoidance. So, we practice poses while communicating: "Face the fear. Nothing lasts forever. Breathe through it."

Remember: experiencing yoga in the midst of an eating disorder may be even harder than teaching it. Be patient (recovery doesn't happen overnight). As teachers, we are the connection to the lesson, encouraging students to open up to the degree they can.

Understanding the disorder is key to understanding recovery. No one chooses to have an eating disorder. Everyone who enters treatment is choosing, at some level, to recover. Embodiment is not an option in recovery; eventually it *has* to happen. That's why yoga is so relevant in treatment.

Conclusion

The future of yoga in treatment is bright. Thanks to modern neuroscience, we have greater ability than ever before to track the "unseen" functions of the mind. With the right kind of research, brain imaging, support and training, I believe yoga will be proven a powerful, efficient, cost-effective (and reimbursable) treatment modality for eating disorders.

Namaste.

19 The Red Tent: Yoga Community in Treatment and Beyond

Caroline Keating

We are complex and awesome beings. Born into a culture that prizes image over substance, it is easy to see why many of us look to the physical body when trying to effect change or exert control in our lives. In this pursuit some of us fall harder than others. Carolyn Costin uses the term "cultural canaries in the coal mine" to describe individuals who, in pursuit of cultural ideals, develop eating disorders. For genetic, psychological and/or other reasons, these individuals are often the most sensitive to our culture's obsession with appearance and its focus on external qualities.

For seven years, I taught yoga to eating disorder clients at Carolyn's Southern California clinic, Monte Nido. There—and elsewhere in our culture—I saw (and still see) women heavy in the heart and soul, disconnected from their bodies. Desperate to heal what Carolyn called "soul-self," they manipulate their physical body and metabolism by restricting, binging and purging their food or compulsively exercising to get and stay thin and in shape.

I have found that their instincts for self-healing are often correct. For instance, many of them *do* need to fast, not from food, but from toxic-media. Acting from intellect they turn to what the culture tells them is wrong: their physical bodies. In reality, change must be enacted on more subtle layers of their being and through a knowing that is more soulful and embodied than intellect. Within a culture that champions intellect it is difficult for women to both find and trust this other kind of knowing. They need the map and the myths that were once received in women's rites of passage but have vanished from our modern cultural landscape.

Even before trying therapy or a treatment program, many women look to yoga to find these missing pieces. Their instincts are right; yoga is rich with practices and mythologies that can fill the void left by our eroding sense of purpose and tradition in modern life. Unfortunately, their instincts are also often impaired, which can be problematic if they embark on a path in yoga without proper guidance.

When loosely applied, yoga philosophy can be co-opted by the very "disordered-self" that each woman in recovery must overcome. I have seen women compulsively perform yogic push-ups, when they really need to condition their funny bone. I see them submit to a torturous form of "self-discipline" by adhering to dogma (about yoga, dieting and a host of other things), when they desperately need to find and follow their wish bone. I see women choose and justify yoga practices of rigid self-abuse over self-empowering practices based on earnest self-inquiry.

Broken in the heart, these women do not quite understand the inherent strength of their soul. They mistakenly pursue "self-mastery" at the expense of their mental and physical well-being. Inappropriately applied, yoga can become a socially acceptable practice of continued illusion and self-injury for women in recovery. It can become a dumping station for the one thing a woman in recovery needs most: her sense of personal power. Yoga can be used to imprison oneself further or find liberation.

When understood and applied appropriately, yoga philosophy can guide a woman through multi-dimensional layers of being to her core essence or soul.

The Panchamaya Kosha Model,[1] of yoga offers a treasure map that modern women are missing from their lives. It outlines how to nourish and heal our whole being by working on and through five layers or Koshas (sheaths), with soul-self nestled in the center: Anamaya Kosha (food/physical body), Pranamaya Kosha (breath body), Manomaya Kosha (mental body), Vijnanamaya Kosha (wisdom body), Anandamaya Kosha (bliss body). Working through the Koshas aligns mind, body and soul. The individual sheaths of this model are sometimes depicted through the imagery of a bird (quite fittingly for the cultural canaries I've worked with). If properly nourished, and with all of its parts in balance and intact, the bird will soar.

I brought this model from India to Monte Nido and watched how learning simple concepts like breath, balance and inner awareness helped women connect with their bodies in a healthy way. I saw balance return to their physical bodies. As is common when midwifing the eating disorder recovery process, I witnessed some women experience a second menarche when their metabolism and hormonal functions restored. The return of menstruation represents a milestone of recovery—yet clients mourn it with comments like: "I'm so fat I got my period." Without a connection to what menstruation represents, they remain prisoners of our cultural con-job: the reframing of a woman's creative power from the blessing that it is into "the curse."

Sadly, our culture does not practice rite of passage rituals or female mentoring that help girls understand and accept this transition into maturity and feminine power. Instead, girls are allowed to believe that menstruation is inconvenient, messy, gross and a sign of having too much body fat. It is something that they should control, minimize or even eliminate. In this and many other ways girls are too often silenced, ridiculed and lose their connection to their natural authentic selves. Many succumb to eating disorders, addiction, depression and other problems.

At Monte Nido, clients who start menstruating are given a ceremony to honor this event as an important rite of passage. The community celebrates both the physical healing and the return of female creative power. This can serve as an initiation into accepting our bodies and authentic selves as sacred.

As a yoga teacher, I am geared to help people see the power of their bodies and the beauty of its function. I wanted to help women with eating disorders see that menstruation's reappearance is an indicator that all the sheaths of their being are coming back into harmony. I wanted to help them get to a point where they could recognize and celebrate this gift. Monte Nido's second menarche ceremonies became the catalyst for raising a red tent. I realized that the Panchamaya Kosha model wasn't complete for women healing the wounds of patriarchy while still living within its confines. Women in recovery need a *sixth* sheath, a female-only sacred space, to keep the toxically wounded outside culture at bay while attending to their healing.

Like many treatment centers, Monte Nido offers a kind of sheath or "safe space" for women. The women are listened to, fed, supported, taught to speak their truth and healed. They are not exposed to popular magazines that contain fashion dos and don'ts, the latest fad diets, and which celebrities have recently gained or lost weight. Cell phone and computer use is limited and even books and television shows have to be approved. There are no full length mirrors and clients are not told their exact weight. This might seem harsh but it provides a space for healing that gives clients a break from (and serves as an antidote for) the cultural forces that play a part in the development and/or maintenance of eating disorders. Clients who first resist such "control," eventually come to understand and appreciate a space and environment conducive to healing body and soul.

I was plagued by the feedback and questions from graduating clients about what happens when women leave treatment and re-enter the mainstream culture. Fresh from the micro-culture of treatment, women often immediately felt the toxic common culture chipping away at them. Many described the urge to lose weight, felt guilty enjoying food, or were enticed to join "calorie burning" yoga classes.

Something became very clear: the sixth sheath, a female-only safe space, is not just important for a woman's recovery but can be essential for any female wanting to thrive amidst the current culture.

Women have instinctually practiced self-care in community for millennia. Historically, women came together in the red tent to attend the major transitions in their lives, birth, menarche, childbearing, menopause and death, as well as tend to the monthly cycle of their fertility years. In addition to preventative self-care, the red tent has long staked its ground in interdependence. It has helped women find the power and reward of taking one's place in a greater community.

Now more than ever women need such a counter-cultural safe house to heal their culturally inflicted traumas. My work with women in recovery convinced me that it was time to resurrect the red tent for all girls and women. I believed that by bringing the red tent back into the social fabric of daily life, not just for recovery but for continued well-being, girls and women would have an on-going opportunity to heal the toxic culture as well as themselves.

Based on this belief I created The Red Tent in Venice, California in 2005. It served in the ways that I had hoped, as a continued supportive space for women after eating disorder treatment as well as an entry point for women who were just beginning to identify their profound dis-ease within common culture. It served in ways that surprised me as I saw women emerging from their own recovery to begin dreaming of a different future for the next generation of girls. We began balancing our efforts in recovery with plans for prevention.

The Red Tent served all women. We began with just a skeleton of a yoga curriculum that offered postures, breathing techniques, contemplative exercises, chanting and ritual designed to work through the Koshas and reconnect women to themselves and the cycles of nature. For instance, in the fall, we fell like leaves, taking our postures to the floor. Contemplative exercises dared us to inquire into our shadow selves. We discussed endings. We chanted in honor of them. We circled up together and felt the safety and comfort of sharing our truths in the simple ritual of a communal talking stick.

Inside the tent women inquired, rested, tended, cried, meditated, moved, occasionally played dead and eventually found a sense of self that many had feared was lost forever. At first, we called this sense of self, "Soul self," "True self," or "authentic self." Then, we just started describing it in detail whenever we spotted it. It enchanted and inspired us like a muse.

Tired of waiting to be kissed awake, these women were ready for an adventure. They wanted to learn navigation of power, trust, surrender, intuition, intimacy and equality. They wanted to reduce their vulnerability to recreating historical patterns, and cycles of abuse.

Women were ripe and ready, stepping off the edge of comfort without a second thought. I remember a woman deeply troubled by her critical inner voices and struggling mightily to silence or overcome them. During a goddess pose (utkata konasana) sequence one day, she suddenly stomped her feet down on the floor with the unabashed, ground-shaking impact of a sumo wrestler. Her entire body radiated liberation as her voice exclaimed: "Fuck it!" to the chorus of self-judgment holding her captive. In that moment, we saw a woman literally step into her power.

Women also experienced their power in new ways through surrender and rest. As they lay in savasana (corpse pose) after a series of yoga postures, I often read a beautiful passage designed to instigate wonder for the body. The overwhelming majority like the first line best:

Your femur is stronger than granite—and it is hollow.

Their love for these words sums up what I saw happening in the room: women experiencing the profound strength that comes from realizing who they really are and the true strength they have. They were learning how to release the life-strangling grip of control and be at ease with their inner life and soul self.

Cycling through the seasonally inspired curriculum, we healed our female soul-selves by seeing the cultural lens that is ever distorting our experience of true-nature. We began leaving that lens, with our shoes, at the door and stopped bothering to pick it back up on the way out. We began focusing on our newly kindled sense of authenticity. It was clear that we were working with fire—women's creative fire, to be exact. I felt the alchemy happening under our humble tent and the reactions created outside of it. We were into something powerful, taboo and incendiary. A naturally arising sense of mystery both spooked and excited us.

Through breath, movement and community, women find the courage to speak our truths. And, we find the endurance to stand in our truths. I remember the morning that I realized: "We are resurrecting a menstrual hut in the middle of Los Angeles!" I laughed out loud. It was absurd. It was important. And it did cause problems in my life:

- The ring of urine someone left around our building perimeter.
- The monthly papering of literature about God's alleged hatred of lesbians.
- The stake hurled through the office window, landing inches from where I sat typing.

Clearly, we were tapping into a cultural nerve (or maybe a cultural vein) with our re-embrace of the female blood mysteries—in essence, the old ways that deem a woman blessed by the very thing we've been duped into thinking is our curse: our bodies' ability to cycle along with all of nature. Embedded in a wounded culture, we were stirring up "trouble" by celebrating a woman's "wise wound."

Even *Yogi Times* magazine headlined an article about us with: "The Red Tent, a place for troubled women." At first, we were incensed. How could a magazine devoted to enlightened living perpetuate the idea that women who embraced their bodies and cycles were troubled? Eventually we saw the light and the humor. The headline was exactly right: we *are all* troubled women. We're deeply troubled by the world around us. We're determined to gather, and do things differently moving forward.

In raising a red tent, I've seen what happens to a woman and to her world when she realizes the awesomeness of her body, when "the curse" of her blood mystery is reclaimed as a blessing. I've seen women move from feeling awful to feeling awe-filled about their bodies. As they step into the most grounded power, the transformation is miraculous. Divine feminine becomes a verb and they begin handcrafting a life with purpose—a life guided from within rather than without.

Of course, even with appropriate initiation, the mysterious gift of our female creative power can leave us questioning: How do we channel our power, if we pick it up at all? Or, will we curse it and walk away? Will we celebrate our natural power or dam(n) it? Will it make us into heroines or bring us to our knees?

I am humbled, sometimes scared, and ever inspired by the women gathered together to do this work of celebrating their bodies, their power, their soul selves, and living authentic lives against all the odds and obstacles imbedded in the current cultural climate. Every one of them is my heroine; my work and life is ever indebted to their courage.

Note

1 Described in Chapter 3.

Index

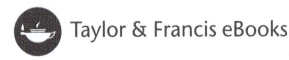

Taylor & Francis eBooks

Helping you to choose the right eBooks for your Library

Add Routledge titles to your library's digital collection today. Taylor and Francis ebooks contains over 50,000 titles in the Humanities, Social Sciences, Behavioural Sciences, Built Environment and Law.

Choose from a range of subject packages or create your own!

Benefits for you

» Free MARC records
» COUNTER-compliant usage statistics
» Flexible purchase and pricing options
» All titles DRM-free.

REQUEST YOUR FREE INSTITUTIONAL TRIAL TODAY

Free Trials Available
We offer free trials to qualifying academic, corporate and government customers.

Benefits for your user

» Off-site, anytime access via Athens or referring URL
» Print or copy pages or chapters
» Full content search
» Bookmark, highlight and annotate text
» Access to thousands of pages of quality research at the click of a button.

eCollections – Choose from over 30 subject eCollections, including:

Archaeology	Language Learning
Architecture	Law
Asian Studies	Literature
Business & Management	Media & Communication
Classical Studies	Middle East Studies
Construction	Music
Creative & Media Arts	Philosophy
Criminology & Criminal Justice	Planning
Economics	Politics
Education	Psychology & Mental Health
Energy	Religion
Engineering	Security
English Language & Linguistics	Social Work
Environment & Sustainability	Sociology
Geography	Sport
Health Studies	Theatre & Performance
History	Tourism, Hospitality & Events

For more information, pricing enquiries or to order a free trial, please contact your local sales team: www.tandfebooks.com/page/sales